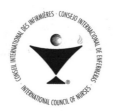

International Council of Nurses
Improving Health through Nursing Research

EDITED BY

WILLIAM L. HOLZEMER, RN, PhD, FAAN

School of Nursing
Rutgers University,
Newark, New Jersey, USA

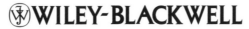

WILEY-BLACKWELL
A John Wiley & Sons, Ltd., Publication

This edition first published 2010
© 2010 The International Council for Nurses (ICN)

Wiley-Blackwell is an imprint of John Wiley & Sons, formed by the merger of Wiley's
global Scientific, Technical and Medical business with Blackwell Publishing.

Registered office
John Wiley & Sons Ltd, The Atrium, Southern Gate, Chichester, West Sussex,
PO19 8SQ, United Kingdom

Editorial offices
9600 Garsington Road, Oxford, OX4 2DQ, United Kingdom
2121 State Avenue, Ames, Iowa 50014-8300, USA

For details of our global editorial offices, for customer services and for information about how to
apply for permission to reuse the copyright material in this book please see our website at
www.wiley.com/wiley-blackwell.

Library of Congress Cataloging-in-Publication Data

Improving health through nursing research / edited by William L. Holzemer. – 1st ed.
  p. ; cm.
Includes bibliographical references and index.
ISBN 978-1-4051-3411-8 (pbk. : alk. paper)
1. Nursing–Research. 2. Evidence-based nursing. I. Holzemer, William L.
II. International Council of Nurses.
[DNLM: 1. Nursing Research. 2. Evidence-Based Nursing. 3. Research Design.
WY 20.5 I345 2009]

RT81.5.I47 2009
610.73072–dc22
2009020416

A catalogue record for this book is available from the British Library.

Set in 10/11.5pt Times NR MT by Graphicraft Limited, Hong Kong
Printed and bound in Malaysia by KHL Printing Co Sdn Bhd

1   2010

Contents

List of Contributors

Lauren S. Aaronson, PhD, RN, FAAN, University of Kansas Medical Center, USA

John Arudo, BSN, MPH, MSc, Aga Khan University, Nairobi, Kenya

Suzanne Bakken, RN, DNSc, Columbia University School of Nursing, USA

Julaluk Baramee, RN, PhD, Burapha University, Chonburi, Thailand

Mary A Blegen, RN, PhD, Center for Patient Safety, School of Nursing, University of California, San Francisco, USA

Flora Cornish, PhD, MSc, BA, Glasgow Caledonian University, UK

Leanne M. Currie, RN, DNSc, Columbia University Department of Biomedical Informatics, USA

Linda Ferguson, BA, Glasgow Caledonian University, UK

Erika Sivarajan Froelicher, RN, MA, MPH, PhD, University of California, San Francisco, USA

Minrie Greeff, BA, MCir, PhD, North-West University, Potchefstroom Campus, South Africa

Sarie Human, DCur, RN, RM, University of South Africa, Pretoria, South Africa

Marjolein M. Iversen, Bergen University College, Norway

Ritamarie John, RN, PNP, DrNP, Columbia University School of Nursing, USA

Jeanne K. Kemppainen, PhD, RN, University of North Carolina, Wilmington, USA

Teri Lindgren, RN, PhD, University of California, San Francisco, USA

Barbara Parfitt, PhD, MSc, McommH, Glasgow Caledonian University, UK

Carmen J. Portillo, RN, PhD, FAAN, University of California, San Francisco, USA

Sally H. Rankin, RN, PhD, FAAN, University of California, San Francisco, USA

William W. Rankin, PhD, Global AIDS Interfaith Alliance, Larkspur, California, USA

Roberta S. Rehm, PhD, RN, University of California, San Francisco, USA

Cornelia Ruland, RN, PhD, Center for Shared Decision Making and Nursing Research, Rikshospitalet University Hospital, Oslo, Norway

Julita Sansoni, RN, PhD, University of Rome, Italy

Kawkab Shishani, RN, PhD, The Hashemite University, Az Zarqa, Jordan

Karen H. Sousa, RN, PhD, Arizona State University, Phoenix, Arizona, USA

Junko Tashiro, RN PhD, St. Luke's College of Nursing, Tokyo, Japan

Leana R. Uys, DSocSc, MSN, BSN, University of KwaZulu-Natal, Durban, South Africa

Dean Wantland, RN, PhD, University of California, San Francisco, USA

June Webber, RN, PhD, Department of International Policy and Development, Canadian Nurses Association, Ottawa, Canada

Suzanne Willard, PhD, CRNP, FAAN, Elizabeth Glaser Pediatric AIDS Foundation, Washington, D.C., USA

Acknowledgments

I would like to thank all of the authors who have contributed their time and valuable expertise to this book. It has been a pleasure to work with them and to help share their many collective years of expertise in nursing research. Thanks also to Yvette Cuca for her support in coordinating work on the book. And I am especially grateful to the book's editor, Paul Engstrom, a San Francisco Bay Area editor and writer who specializes in medicine and health.

Preface

Authors in many parts of the world and I take great pleasure in presenting this introductory textbook, *Improving Health Through Nursing Research*, published by the International Council of Nurses and Wiley-Blackwell. More than two dozen authors contributed, donating their time to support the work of ICN, which will use all proceeds from the book to further the council's mission.

This book is a bit different from traditional introductory texts about nursing research. Some sections you may expect, others you may not.

Part 1 offers a global perspective on health and nursing. As an introduction to the philosophy of science, which builds on knowledge, it addresses some of the topics currently under discussion in nursing about nursing science and theory.

Part 2 builds a case for the mission of nurse scientists: to improve the lives of the individuals, families, and communities we serve. As scientists, our research focuses on improving patient care, enhancing care delivery, building the profession of nursing, and asking research questions that can potentially build evidence for practice.

Part 3 is an introductory overview of quantitative research methods, including experimental design, sampling, instruments, research designs, critique of research, and the preparation and analysis of data. The chapters are purposely not as detailed as those in some texts; rather, they seek to make readers intelligent consumers of published research and to foster the use of research findings in nursing practice.

Part 4 provides an introductory overview of major issues and strategies related to qualitative research methods, including the preparation of textual data for analysis and interpretative methods. These chapters seek to pique readers' interest in learning more about the details of qualitative research methodologies.

Part 5 focuses on processes related to conducting research in clinical and academic settings. Topics include writing a research proposal, managing a study, presenting and publishing findings, and facilitating research. With the tremendous interest in nursing research, we feel it is important to understand what is necessary to conduct and support research in either of these settings.

The two exciting chapters in Part 6 address the translation of research findings into practice. The first chapter links nursing research to informatics and the electronic health record as a data source for capturing variables of interest to nurse scientists. It discusses the technological infrastructure that supports evidence-based practice. The final chapter looks at the many challenges of implementing evidence-based practice in the clinical practice setting.

It I hoped that this book will not only be a fun read, but also launch your journey into a greater understanding of nursing science and help you develop research skills. We also hope it will inspire you to think about clinical practice from both the clinician and scientist perspectives. Enjoy.

William L. Holzemer, RN, PhD, FAAN
Editor

Part 1
Nursing science and global health

Chapter 1
Global perspectives on health and nursing

Barbara Parfitt, Flora Cornish &
Linda Ferguson

Introduction

Health, illness, and health care are global issues requiring global solutions. 'Globalization' is more than a cliché describing abstract economic and political processes. It also has a concrete impact on health and the provision of health care, and suggests that people everywhere are connected. An outbreak of severe acute respiratory syndrome in China is of concern not only to China's neighbors, but also to governments around the world. When a nurse emigrates from Kenya to take up a better paying job caring for the aged in the UK, it affects the workforce and delivery of services in both countries.

This chapter introduces the global priorities for health and health care, and the international organizations – particularly nursing organizations – that coordinate the world community's response to health challenges. Rapid changes in such challenges mean that current tools and mechanisms for health promotion and care will not always be sufficient. High-quality and continuous nursing research is necessary to determine the best ways to promote health and deliver care.

Global priorities for health

Because health problems and health services vary greatly, international organizations and governments have sought to establish common goals and priorities. Such goals ensure that efforts by a wide range of health agencies are appropriately

3

targeted to areas where they can have the greatest impact and that these efforts are coordinated. While there are various ways to establish global priorities, the two approaches discussed here are the Millennium Development Goals and Global Burden of Disease statistics. Priorities concern specific health conditions and the means of addressing them – for example, developing a health care workforce and putting research findings into practice.

Millennium Development Goals

These goals set the agenda for global development efforts from 2000 to 2015. The eight Millennium Development Goals (MDGs) (Box 1.1) were a product of the United Nations' Millennium Summit, which convened in September 2000 to address the role of the UN in the 21st century.[1] Their purpose is to provide a clear framework for all stakeholders involved in pursuing development in developing countries. The goals shape efforts in every setting. Governments and international organizations, including the World Bank, the Organization for Economic Co-operation and Development, and the International Monetary Fund, use them to guide their policies and programs.

All of the MDGs have major implications for health issues, given that economic, social, natural, and political environments are powerful determinants of a population's health. Three of the MDGs – to reduce child mortality, improve maternal health, and combat HIV/AIDS, malaria, and other diseases – are specifically related to health and to the work of nurses and midwives. Each is associated with a set of quantitative, time-bound targets to provide clear aims and allow monitoring of progress (Table 1.1).

Nurses and midwives have much to contribute to achieving the targets. When children die in developing countries, it is usually from preventable or easily treated conditions such as measles, diarrheal diseases, or malaria (United Nations 2006; World Health Organization [WHO] 2003b[2]). Children in poor rural households suffer disproportionately. Nurses have an important role in vaccination because they increase parents' ability to protect children's health, make referrals when necessary, and provide care. A key way to prevent maternal deaths during delivery is to have a skilled attendant, such as a nurse, on hand (United Nations 2006). Nurses' health promotion skills are also crucial in reducing the incidence of HIV/AIDS, malaria, tuberculosis, and other infectious diseases.

Box 1.1: Millennium Development Goals

- Eradicate extreme poverty
- Achieve universal primary education
- Promote gender equality and empower women
- Reduce child mortality
- Improve maternal health
- Combat HIV/AIDS, malaria, and other diseases
- Ensure environmental sustainability
- Develop a global partnership for development

Source: devdata.worldbank.org/gmis/mdg/list_of_goals.htm

Table 1.1 Targets for health-related Millennium Development Goals.

Goal	Target
Reduce child mortality	Reduce by two-thirds among children younger than 5 between 1990 and 2015
Improve maternal health	Reduce maternal mortality ratio by three-quarters between 1990 and 2015
Combat HIV/AIDS, malaria, and other diseases	• Halt HIV/AIDS and begin to reverse their spread by 2015 • Halt malaria and other major diseases and begin to reverse their incidence by 2015

Source: devdata.worldbank.org/gmis/mdg/list_of_goals.htm

To achieve the MDGs, corrective measures focus on public health and primary health care – namely, using well-established methods to prevent health problems. These are not high-tech, crisis interventions; rather, they are simple, community-based services delivered by a skilled health care worker. An appropriate system for distributing medicines and equipment, and an appropriate team to receive referrals when necessary, support these efforts.

Research is needed to determine how best to deliver optimal prevention and health care services using the limited resources available in developing countries. To support the emphasis on primary care and public health, such research should include studies of behaviour change, community participation, and mobilization, and the appropriate configuration of health service teams and community-based models of service delivery.

The MDGs were designed to advance development, as it is broadly understood, in low- and middle-income countries; health is not their primary focus. The health-related goals – child and maternal health, and communicable diseases – target areas in which huge discrepancies exist between developing and developed countries. Other health issues emerge when the topic is the Global Burden of Disease.

Global Burden of Disease

This term describes the biggest health problems around the world. National statistics are used to identify the most common causes of death and the major causes of disability in low, middle, and high-income countries, and to produce a composite measure of disability-adjusted life years (DALYs). DALYs are a gauge of the number of years of healthy life lost because of premature death and disability (Mathers & Loncar 2006). The measure reveals which diseases and risks cause the most problems. Table 1.2 lists, in descending order, the 10 leading causes of the Global Burden of Disease in 2001, the most recent year for which data have been analyzed.

The 10 leading causes include the communicable diseases that have recently been associated with developing countries (for example, diarrheal diseases and malaria) and the non-communicable, chronic conditions (sometimes called 'diseases of modernity,' including depressive disorders, heart disease, and chronic obstructive pulmonary disease [COPD]) that are more typically associated with affluent and aging populations in developed countries.

Table 1.2 The 10 leading causes of the Global Burden of Disease.

Cause	Total DALYs (%)
Perinatal conditions	5.9
Lower respiratory infections	5.6
Ischemic heart disease	5.5
Cerebrovascular disease	4.7
HIV/AIDS	4.7
Diarrheal diseases	3.9
Unipolar depressive disorders	3.4
Malaria	2.6
Chronic obstructive pulmonary disease	2.5
Tuberculosis	2.3

DALY, disability-adjusted life year.
Source: Mathers et al. (2006).

In wealthy countries, chronic conditions have the highest health priority and often are related to an aging population and lifestyle. In the UK and the USA, for example, top priorities are regular exercise, healthy eating, reducing tobacco and alcohol use, and support for good mental health. Much can be done to prevent lifestyle-related illness and disability, although health care expenditures have traditionally focused on treatment rather than prevention. To support nurses' efforts in this regard, a priority should be high-quality research on developing sound and appropriate approaches to health promotion.

However, wealthy countries are not the only ones with aging populations. Between 2000 and 2050, the number of people in the world who are aged 60 years or older will more than triple to 2 billion from 600 million; most of this increase is occurring in developing countries (WHO 2007a). Demographic changes such as these, and improvements in dealing with communicable disease, will have major impacts on the global burden of disease everywhere. Table 1.3 shows what the 10 leading causes of DALYs are projected to be in 2030.

Table 1.3 The 10 leading causes of DALYs by 2030 (projected).

High-income countries	Middle-income countries	Low-income countries
1. Unipolar depressive disorders	1. HIV/AIDS	1. HIV/AIDS
2. Ischemic heart disease	2. Unipolar depressive disorders	2. Perinatal conditions
3. Alzheimer's and other dementias	3. Cerebrovascular disease	3. Unipolar depressive disorders
4. Alcohol use disorders	4. Ischemic heart disease	4. Traffic accidents
5. Diabetes mellitus	5. COPD	5. Ischemic heart disease
6. Cerebrovascular disease	6. Traffic accidents	6. Lower respiratory infections
7. Hearing loss (adult onset)	7. Violence	7. Diarrheal diseases
8. Trachea/bronchus/lung cancer	8. Vision disorders (age-related)	8. Cerebrovascular disease
9. Osteoarthritis	9. Hearing loss (adult onset)	9. Cataracts
10. COPD	10. Diabetes mellitus	10. Malaria

COPD, chronic obstructive pulmonary disease.
Source: Mathers & Loncar (2006).

As developing countries make progress against communicable diseases, they will also have to reorient health services to meet the needs of their aging populations to prevent or delay the onset of age-related conditions, and offer supportive, continuous management of chronic diseases (WHO 2007a). The global changes in demographics and health profiles will necessitate relevant, practice-focused research to establish the most effective ways of dealing with new challenges, such as chronic disease management in resource-poor settings.

Health systems and the health care workforce

Perhaps more important than individual diseases are the health systems and health care workforces necessary to respond to them effectively. Addressing workforce shortages was the focus of the World Health Organization's 2006 World Health Report, which estimated that in order to provide the essential interventions necessary to meet the health-related MDGs, the world needs 2.4 million more doctors, nurses, and midwives. The largest proportional shortfalls are in sub-Saharan Africa and in South and South-East Asia (WHO 2006).

Given the aging of populations and the pressures on health budgets globally, governments are looking for ways to deliver health care more efficiently. They are seeking to reduce costly hospital stays and to deal with health issues in homes and communities as much as possible. Thus, the worldwide focus is moving toward public health and primary care, with an emphasis on family health care programs rather than acute care (Crisp 2007). The favored training approach is to give health care workers the particular skills ('know how') they will need in the community, in contrast to today's primary competency ('know all'). It encourages training in the practice setting, learning from role models, and using problem-solving techniques (WHO 2006). But this approach also poses a danger: producing health care workers who have received inexpensive, low-level training when the developing world needs highly competent professionals who can take responsibility for a broad range of practice and adapt to changing circumstances.

National and international programs have often strived to involve communities in their own health-related decisions, a central concept in the Declaration of Alma-Ata issued 30 years ago at the International Conference on Primary Health Care (WHO 1978). The response to and success of engaging communities with local health care providers have been mixed, although there is evidence that this approach does instill positive and sustainable health behaviours. However, the meaning of 'community' and whether a community is truly participating in health efforts are matters of debate (Midgley et al. 1986).

One key problem for nations is the migration of health care workers. The World Health Report concluded that migration is largely due to the perception among workers of better financial prospects elsewhere. Others fear violence in their home country or see little or no opportunity for career advancement, further education, or satisfactory working conditions (WHO 2006).

The positive and negative impacts of migration are extensive (Kingma 2006). On the positive side, money that workers abroad send home can benefit the local economy. The Philippines, for example, invests in nurse education with the expectation that an oversupply of nurses will venture overseas and send money back to their families. In addition, health care workers may gain skills and expertise in a foreign country that ultimately could benefit their home country when they return. On the negative side, a country loses its investment in the education and preparation of health professionals when they remain abroad, and its own health services may suffer if there is a shortage of qualified workers.

Efforts to manage migration are targeted to both source countries and recipient countries. The former are advised to adjust training so it meets internal workforce needs first and to improve local pay and opportunities for career advancement. Recipient countries are encouraged to foster fair treatment of migrant workers, adopt responsible recruitment policies, and partially compensate source countries for their investment in health professional education (WHO 2006).

Finally, developing an appropriately skilled workforce of professionals for global health requires not only high-quality research on how best to accomplish this, but also mechanisms for sharing expertise in effective health care delivery and bringing research findings into practice. The latter is critical because '[a]pplying what we know already will have a bigger impact on health and disease than any drug or technology likely to be introduced in the next decade' (Pang et al. 2006, p. 284). Effective measles vaccines, bed nets to prevent malaria, and regular physical activity are well-established ways to improve health, but their impact may be limited because implementation is not universal. Research that investigates the best way to turn health knowledge into effective, patient-centered, feasible, and sustainable health care practice is crucial.

Nurses have a major role in delivering services, given that they constitute 80% of the global health care workforce. But they could also play a major research role in innovations and evaluating processes that put knowledge to work. Key areas warranting nursing-related research are the link between education and effective practice, and the practical skills nurses must have to meet the world's health care needs. This research focus requires qualitative research training, beyond quantitative methodologies, because complex health situations in the real world require a broader perspective.

Nurse researchers with sound qualitative skills have an opportunity to inform both the policy and practice of international health development. Lorenz (2007) believes that researchers' current view of global health issues is at risk of becoming detached from daily realities, and suggests that sharing practical experience and success stories by means of critical incident reporting may be a good way to confront health challenges on the national and international levels.

Participating in research aimed at international health issues calls for an understanding of how organizations around the world contribute to that effort and of nurses' important role.

International organizations and development aid

International organizations have never been so important. In addition to providing financial aid, they help integrate services, promote health, and, through research and evaluation, foster expansion of the evidence base for health care practice.

However, coordination of global aid is becoming increasingly complex, largely because of the many organizations now involved in overseas projects.

The average number of donor organizations per country rose to 32 in the 2001–2005 period from 12 in the 1960s. This has caused fragmentation of donor funding and delivery of health services, which may make it difficult for a country receiving aid to use it effectively. Many projects focus vertically on a single health issue, excluding other related and important issues (International Development Association 2007), or on a particular geographic area, such that surrounding areas do not benefit.

Organizations realize they are less likely to achieve desired outcomes if they work alone. Success in education, research, and improved health requires partnerships between developed and developing nations, between donor agencies and the governments receiving their assistance, and between organizations.

The many types of international organizations that contribute to health-related projects are described below.

Voluntary organizations

Private voluntary organizations that support health development date back hundreds of years. For many centuries, religious organizations of all faiths have provided medical and nursing care to the needy and destitute through charitable offerings. Many secular organizations, motivated by humanistic and social concerns, sponsor philanthropic care programs.

These growing independent, non-governmental organizations (NGOs) have contributed to the construction of hospitals and hospices, orphanages, and sanctuaries for lepers, outcasts, and the homeless, and often are the main source of consistent, high-quality care in developing nations. They partner with governments and other organizations. Increasingly, a substantial portion of their funding comes from government and inter-government sources.

Such organizations, which include Oxfam,[3] Save the Children Fund,[4] Christian Aid,[5] Tear Fund,[6] World Vision,[7] Muslim Aid,[8] and Islamic Relief,[9] are dedicated to combating health inequalities and fighting poverty and injustice around the world. They rely on donations and grants from individuals and government sources, frequently provide limited funding for research and scholarship activities, and use volunteers. Immediate problems in communities throughout the developed and developing world could not be addressed without their aid.

Foundations

Large foundations, whose objectives are different from those of NGOs, often fund major development projects, although over the course of many years they also have supported academic courses and fellowships for physicians, dentists, nurses, and technicians. In addition, they provide population and demographic statistics for public health purposes, deliver family planning services, and work to reduce maternal mortality.

These entities include the:

- W.K. Kellogg Foundation,[10] which supports social inclusion and health projects;
- Milbank Memorial Fund,[11] which seeks to improve health by influencing health policy and decision-making;
- Pathfinder International,[12] which supports high-quality family planning and reproductive health services;

- William and Flora Hewlett Foundation,[13] which focuses primarily on solving social and environmental problems;
- Carnegie Foundation for the Advancement of Teaching[14];
- Ford Foundation,[15] a resource that people worldwide can tap in efforts to instill democracy, reduce poverty and injustice, promote international co-operation, and advance human achievement;
- Rockefeller Foundation,[16] which addresses the root causes of serious problems in the world and establishes partnerships to overcome them. One of its major contribution is the development and distribution of vaccines in developing countries;
- Bill & Melinda Gates Foundation.[17] This tries to reduce inequalities in the USA and elsewhere through programs that seek solutions to poverty, hunger, and disease. The foundation recognizes that there is very little research on ways to prevent or cure some of the world's biggest killers, such as malaria and tuberculosis; and the
- Aga Khan Foundation.[18] This supports social development in low-income countries.

Large corporate foundations do not typically accept grant applications from individuals. Rather, they work with tax-exempt organizations in developed countries.

Two trusts worth mentioning are the Wellcome Trust,[19] which supports medical and health-related projects primarily through research, as well as medical students and medical personnel, and the Nuffield Trust,[20] which seeks to improve health care quality primarily in the UK. However, its international portfolio includes European and other countries.

Private industry

Although pharmaceutical companies make a major contribution to international health, their role is controversial. Historically, they have been heavily criticized for putting profit above the needs of the developing world and for producing medications and medical supplies that meet the needs of their own regions and that generate profits and enough revenue to fund research and development. This issue is very complex, however, in part because drugmakers provide employment and investment in the developing and mid-developing world, and because the research they conduct may or may not ultimately benefit all patients globally. Johnson & Johnson[21] is among the companies that adhere to self-established ethical principles, including meeting its responsibilities to customers, employees, and the community.

The World Health Assembly, a WHO governing entity, resolved in 1975 that essential medicines should be reasonably priced and of good quality, and should correspond to countries' particular health needs (WHO 2000). In subsequent years, the WHO (1988) identified indicators for monitoring countries' progress toward developing a drug policy. It also defined 'essential medicines' and recommended using those that are effective against prevalent diseases and cost-effective, and ensuring their availability, quality, and appropriateness (WHO 2002).

Despite these efforts, an estimated 25% of medicines in developing countries are counterfeit (they contain altered or imitated active and inactive ingredients which may be harmful) or substandard (WHO 2003a). Other problems include outdated medicines and drugs that have been tampered with for resale at higher profit. The International Council of Nurses (2005) cites a number of counterfeiting incidents worldwide that have led to many deaths. There is a need for further investigation and research to assess the full impact of counterfeit and substandard medicines in developing nations.

Some pharmaceutical companies actively discourage the misuse of drugs, fight counterfeiting, and strive to improve drug quality. Merck,[22] for example, says it is a research-driven company that puts patients first. A central theme in its mission statement is promoting innovation to improve customers' quality of life. In addition, Merck has set high ethical standards for itself.

The main objective of the International Federation of Pharmaceutical Manufacturers and Associations,[23] a non-profit NGO, is to promote therapeutic and preventative medical innovations, and to foster collaborations among international organizations, especially those working in developing countries.

Government and inter-government agencies

These entities are critical because they ensure a degree of coordination between donors and recipients. The Organization for Economic Co-operation and Development (OECD), for example, is a major player which shares its expertise with 70 countries worldwide, analyzing the impact of globalization and national policies on economic development and growth. It provides statistical and economic data that member countries can use in responding to challenges. OECD's 30 government members produce 60% of the world's goods, and embrace democracy and market-based economies. Its operational unit is the Development Co-operation Directorate, which seeks to create and sustain economic growth and stability. The OECD does not allocate resources; rather, it participates in negotiations on a framework for international cooperation and corporate governance of aid provided by its members through the Development Co-operation Directorate.

OECD members have their own agencies for distributing funds overseas. Among them are the Department for International Development in the UK, the United States Agency for International Development, the Canadian International Development Agency, the Danish International Development Agency, the Swedish International Development Cooperation Agency, the Norwegian Agency for Development Cooperation, and the Japan International Cooperation Agency. Between 1990 and 1998, OECD members' share of international aid fell from 0.09% to 0.05% (United Nations Conference on Trade and Development 2000).

The World Bank,[24] whose members include 185 countries and five associate organizations, is a vital source of financial aid and technical advice. One of its members, the International Development Association, targets the poorest countries. Loans the association makes on favorable terms seek to reduce population growth and poverty, enhance governance and the investment climate, and develop physical and human infrastructures. Global health is not a priority for the World Bank, but the bank has become increasingly involved in WHO-associated health projects. The key health issue, it believes, is the need to bolster health systems. It has also called for a major effort to strengthen financial commitments from potential donors so health-related aid can make the MDGs achievable. This requires that a sound regulatory framework for private–public collaboration, good governance–insurance schemes, trained health personnel, and a basic health service infrastructure be in place to ensure equitable health, nutrition, and appropriate provision of care.

The WHO is the UN's specialized agency for coordinating international health. It is governed by 193 member states through the World Health Assembly, which sets health priorities and adopts resolutions. The WHO's six core functions are leading international health efforts, shaping the world health research agenda, establishing norms and standards, articulating policy based on ethical evidence, providing technical support, and monitoring health trends.

Like other international organizations, the WHO operates in an increasingly complex, and constantly and rapidly changing, world. Among its many activities are:

- Promoting development, reducing poverty, and encouraging policies for equal access to health resources and equal provision of health services, especially among disadvantaged and vulnerable populations;
- Fostering health security, given the increasing and ever-present threat of global epidemics;
- Strengthening health-related human resources;
- Promoting adequate health financing and evidence-based practice in the development and strengthening of health systems;
- Enhancing partnerships with other UN agencies and international organizations;
- Encouraging collaboration among entities, given the fragmentation of efforts; and
- Improving performance. For example, the WHO encourages adequately funded work environments that support and motivate staff, and that are managed based on results, which is critical for effective and efficient reforms.[25]

The WHO's member states recognize that nursing and midwifery are an important component – one that needs to be strengthened so it contributes effectively to improving health outcomes. The organization's efforts to bolster that component, which stem from numerous World Health Assembly resolutions,[26] include formulating policies and offering technical advice that promote capacity building, and establishing collaborations. It encourages research-based evidence to inform effective decision-making.

Another UN organization is the United Nations Children's Fund (UNICEF).[27] Unlike the WHO, UNICEF relies entirely on voluntary contributions for funding. Much of its work focuses on controlling infectious diseases such as tuberculosis, leprosy, malaria, and HIV/AIDS in children; providing clean drinking water; educating children; and delivering maternal and child health services. Per UN mandate, UNICEF advocates children's rights by ensuring that their basic needs are met and that they have opportunities to reach their full potential. UNICEF also has a special mandate to protect the rights of women and girls, including full participation in political, social, and economic development.

A means for nurses to contribute to the international health agenda is the WHO's Collaborating Centres for Nursing and Midwifery Development.[28] Nearly 40 centers worldwide provide knowledge and technical expertise; are often involved in innovative practices and research projects to facilitate technical cooperation; foster an exchange of information, expertise, and experience between developing countries; and contribute to national efforts to improve health outcomes. One of the collaborating centers' strengths is their links to, and partnerships with, national and international institutions and ministries of health.

In January 2000, the WHO's executive board urged member states to take full advantage of the centers' resources and services, and to expand their own capacity for training, research, and collaboration. It also urged the centers to build working relationships with each other and national institutions recognized by the WHO – in particular, by establishing or joining collaborative networks with support from the WHO. Indeed, the centers have formed an independent global network that aims to pool all of their strengths and achieve key international goals in research, education, and development.

International nursing organizations

As a federation of national nurse associations, the International Council of Nurses (ICN),[29] founded in 1899, is an entity operated by and for nurses, representing nurses in more than 128 countries. It is the world's first and widest-reaching international organization for health professionals. The ICN promotes quality nursing care for all, sound health policies, research, the advancement of nursing knowledge to improve standards of care, respect for the profession, and a competent and satisfied workforce. Importantly, the council does more than bring nurses together and move them and their profession forward; it also influences health policy. It achieves these goals through partnerships and strategic alliances with government agencies, NGOs, and other organizations.

An organization that also contributes to the research and development agenda is Sigma Theta Tau International,[30] a nursing honor society. It promotes scholarship excellence by admitting honorary members from the entire academic spectrum. Elsewhere, the European Academy of Nursing Science,[31] whose members have made significant contributions to their field, supports PhD students and meets regularly to share expertise. Although the academy focuses on Europe, it does seek to influence, through research and scientific endeavor, nursing-related international issues.

Conclusions

A broad view of international development efforts reveals a number of important themes:

- Organizations respond to global health needs in a variety of ways;
- The fragmented nature of global health care is a source of great concern because it squanders valuable human and financial resources;
- Countries in the northern hemisphere do not provide sufficient aid to enable meaningful change;
- Large institutions such as the WHO and the World Bank drive policies regarding the development of health care systems; and
- Nurses have an important role in providing evidence-based research which helps inform and influence international policy and practice.

While the international contribution that nursing makes to research and health care development is weak compared to medicine's, nurses nevertheless have an essential role in promoting and sustaining community health. They are key protagonists in improving access to services and fostering community participation.

However, two noteworthy trends are the shift in delivery of services from the primary care model of the 1970s and 1980s to a vertical, specialized approach, and the replacement of nurses with other health care workers. In addition to creating gaps in health care, these trends could reduce the nursing workforce, even though the global human resource crisis cited by the WHO (2006) clearly warrants an increase. Because nurses have wide-ranging expertise and, from a research perspective, recognize the importance of holistic care, they may be best suited to tackle international health problems.

There is an urgent need for research that evaluates and reveals the impact of nursing care on the health of developed and developing countries. Without it, the nursing profession as it is known today could vanish.

Notes

1   www.un.org/millennium
2   www.who.int/whr/2003/chapter1/en/index2.html
3   www.oxfam.org.uk
4   www.savethechildren.org
5   www.christian-aid.org.uk
6   www.tearfund.org
7   www.worldvision.org.uk
8   www.muslimaid.org
9   www.islamic-relief.com
10   www.wkkf.org
11   www.milbank.org
12   www.pathfind.org
13   www.hewlett.org
14   www.carnegiefoundation.org
15   www.fordfound.org
16   www.rockfound.org
17   www.Gatesfoundation.org
18   www.akdn.org/agency/akf.html
19   www.wellcome.ac.uk
20   www.nuffieldtrust.org.uk
21   www.jnj.com
22   www.merck.com/cr/company
23   ifpma.org/About-Us/about.aspx
24   www.worldbank.org
25   www.who.int/about/agenda/en/index.html
26   WHA42.27, WHA45.5, WHA47.9, WHA48.8, WHA54.12, WHA59.23, and WHA59.27.
27   www.unicef.org
28   www.whocc.gcal.ac.uk
29   www.icn.ch
30   www.nursingsociety.org/default.aspx
31   www.european-academy-of-nursing-science.com

References

Crisp, N. (2007) *Global health partnerships: The UK contribution to health in developing countries.* London: COI.

International Council of Nurses (2005) *Counterfeits kill: Nurses target counterfeit medicines.* Geneva: International Council of Nurses.

International Development Association (2007) *An architecture: An overview of the main trends in official development assistance flows.* Resource Mobilization Department (FRM). Geneva: World Bank.

Kingma, M. (2006) *Nurses on the move: Migration and the global health care economy.* Ithaca, New York: Cornell University Press.

Lorenz, N. (2007) Effectiveness of global health partnerships: Will the past repeat itself? *Bulletin of the World Health Organization* **85**(7), 587. Geneva: WHO.

Mathers, C.D. & Loncar, D. (2006) Projections of global mortality and burden of disease from 2002 to 2030. *PLoS Medicine* **3**(11), 2011–2030.

Mathers, C.D., Lopez, A.D. & Murray, C.J.L. (2006) The burden of disease and mortality by condition: Data, methods, and results for 2001. In A.D. Lopez, C.D. Mathers, M. Ezzati, et al. (Eds) *Global burden of disease and risk factors* (pp. 45–240). New York: Oxford University Press.

Midgley, J., Hall, A., Hardiman, M. & Dhanpaul, N. (1986) *Community participation, social development, and the state.* London: Methuen & Co.

Pang, T., Gray, M. & Evans, T. (2006) The 15th grand challenge for global public health. *Lancet* **367**(9507), 284–286.

United Nations (2006) *The Millennium Development Goals report 2006.* New York: United Nations.

United Nations Conference on Trade and Development (2000) *The least developed countries 2000 report.* New York: United Nations.

World Health Organization (1978) *Health for all by the year 2000.* Geneva: WHO.

World Health Organization (1988) *Guidelines for developing national drug policies.* Geneva: WHO.

World Health Organization (2000) *The use of essential drugs. Eighth report of the WHO expert committee*, WHO Technical Report Series No. 882. Geneva: WHO.

World Health Organization (2002) *The selection and use of essential medicines. Report of the WHO expert committee.* Geneva: WHO.

World Health Organization (2003a) *Substandard and counterfeit medicines*, Fact Sheet No. 275. Geneva: WHO.

World Health Organization (2003b) *The world health report 2003: Shaping the future.* Geneva: WHO.

World Health Organization (2006) *The world health report 2006: Working together for health.* Geneva: WHO.

World Health Organization (2007a) *What are the public health implications of global aging?* Geneva: WHO.

Chapter 2
Building knowledge

Sally H. Rankin & William W. Rankin

Knowledge development in science

Nursing became a structured discipline in the late 19th century when Florence Nightingale began codifying and formalizing nursing knowledge. Ever since, research that relies on building theories through induction and deduction for the purpose of testing hypotheses has influenced nursing science (Figure 2.1).

Both induction and deduction are scientific processes, and both are appropriate in advancing different kinds of knowledge, usually through research. The nursing, person, environment, and health domains in the 'nursing meta-paradigm,' first described in the 1980s, have been criticized as either too restrictive or no longer pertinent to the development of knowledge (Holmes & Gastaldo 2004). Yet the paradigm still is a useful heuristic device because it shows how philosophy, science, and theory are integrated. A given research approach depends heavily on the philosophy from which conceptual models are derived.

Early philosophical thought

Philosophical thought apparently began sometime between 800 and 200 BC when the Greeks joined the Hebrew prophets, Lao-Tzu and Confucius in China, Zarathustra in Turkey, and Buddha in India in thinking about the world. The Greeks traveled widely, were sophisticated writers and artists (especially in architecture), and had a fairly stable government. Their earliest philosophers tried to understand the world without reference to Greece's polytheistic culture. They also tried to separate explanations of physical phenomena from God and magic – asking, for example, why the sun rises and sets, what the Earth is made of, and why metals are hard.

The Greek philosophers realized that physical objects – trees, water, human beings – are always changing and wanted to learn universal truths about them. This was the first attempt to gather data. Data gained from sensory experience

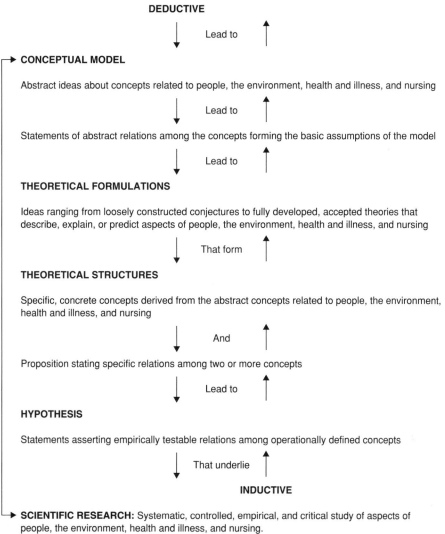

PHILOSOPHY: Nursing is concerned with statements of beliefs and values about individuals, families and groups, their environment, their health and illness, and the practice of nursing

DEDUCTIVE

Lead to

CONCEPTUAL MODEL

Abstract ideas about concepts related to people, the environment, health and illness, and nursing

Lead to

Statements of abstract relations among the concepts forming the basic assumptions of the model

Lead to

THEORETICAL FORMULATIONS

Ideas ranging from loosely constructed conjectures to fully developed, accepted theories that describe, explain, or predict aspects of people, the environment, health and illness, and nursing

That form

THEORETICAL STRUCTURES

Specific, concrete concepts derived from the abstract concepts related to people, the environment, health and illness, and nursing

And

Proposition stating specific relations among two or more concepts

Lead to

HYPOTHESIS

Statements asserting empirically testable relations among operationally defined concepts

That underlie

INDUCTIVE

SCIENTIFIC RESEARCH: Systematic, controlled, empirical, and critical study of aspects of people, the environment, health and illness, and nursing.

Figure 2.1 From philosophy to scientific research. After Fawcett (1984).
Source: Adapted from Fawcett, 1984.

is empirical data and knowledge based on it is empiricism, the basis of science and scientific methods.

As the early philosophers were attempting to comprehend the world, the sophists, another Greek philosophical group, emerged and sought to understand people and why they behaved the way they did. In this pursuit, the sophists accumulated a broad range of facts for use in formulating arguments.

Socrates developed his philosophy in opposition to the sophists, who had abandoned their search for objective truth in favor of rhetorical skill. He was interested in morality, ethics, justice, truth, and goodness. Plato, a student of Socrates, founded the academy where Aristotle later studied for 20 years. Plato's focus was knowledge, which he defined as an interaction between the perceiver and the perceived under the guidance of the soul or the mind. In his view, people perceive imperfect copies of things in the ideal world. For example, the image of a chair represents another, more perfect chair as it would be in the ideal world.

Aristotle founded a school in Athens known as the Lyceum. At the time, it was referred to as the 'peripatetic school' because Aristotle walked as he taught. He differentiated three realms of thinking, but did not distinguish philosophy from science, as people do today. The realms were:

(1) The first philosophy or science, which included physics and mathematics;
(2) The practical sciences, which encompassed ethics, economics, and political science; and
(3) The productive sciences, which included disciplines such as the fine arts, medicine, architecture, and rhetoric (Losee 2001).

Aristotle's contribution to nursing science was his attempt to classify knowledge. He did this through a form of deductive reasoning called the syllogism, which relies on a premise to develop a conclusion and is the basic building block of argument even today. An example of a syllogism is: All men are mortal. Plato is a man. Therefore, Plato is mortal.

By means of induction, Aristotle used his observations of the world to formulate explanatory principles. Deduction then led him back to more observations. Thus, induction is the process of generating a universal conclusion by observing particulars. Deduction is the opposite – reasoning from the general to the specific. According to Aristotle, a conclusion drawn inductively should have the status of a universal law. However, because it is impossible to scrutinize every instance of something, induction cannot generate scientific proofs. The only way to do that is through syllogisms.

Claims to knowledge based on induction or deduction had to be irrefutable in order to qualify as absolute truth. The end-product of these procedures came to be called science. The notion that science is systematic, objective, and truth-seeking germinated from Aristotle's work.

The search for knowledge fostered attempts to uncover the 'essence' of things. For example, what is the essence of an animal, of caring? According to Aristotle, when the essence of something has been determined, one can claim to have discovered its fundamental identity. This commitment became the basis for the philosophical school of thought called 'essentialism.' Essential properties are those that a thing cannot lose without ceasing to exist. Once the essence is found, the 'cause' of a thing is ascertained (Ladyman 2002). Plato believed, for instance, that the 'soul' animated the body, and that without it, a living being could no longer exist.

Aristotle's *Metaphysics* included the idea that 'nature does not act without a goal.' He ascribed goals to physics, biology, and ethics. Today, it is difficult to ascribe a goal to physics, although that task may be easier in the realms of biology or ethics. This notion became the basis of Roman Catholic doctrine that the goal of sexual intercourse is the production of offspring and that any other goal of coition, such as sexual pleasure alone, is wrong.

The major contributions of Aristotle to the philosophy of nursing science include inductive and deductive processes, and the construction of taxonomies for the purpose of gaining knowledge. Charles Darwin developed his taxonomies based on Aristotelian classifications, and taxonomies for nursing diagnoses and interventions conform with them. Aristotle's philosophy – passed down through St. Thomas Aquinas, the Italian Dominican friar and writer who lived in the 13th century – included the unenlightened notion that women are 'unfinished men.' His views about women held sway throughout the Middle Ages; they influenced Christian church doctrine and, therefore, social views in general.

Modern philosophy and its influence on science

René Descartes, a 17th century French philosopher, mathematician, and scientist, is known as the father of modern philosophy. He believed that rationalism, or reason, is the source of all knowledge. In 1619, Descartes had three dreams that led him to believe he had been called to reconstruct human knowledge so it would embody the certainty expressed only in mathematics. He used a deductive hierarchy of propositions rather than induction. According to his theory of scientific method, an experimenter must provide knowledge of the conditions under which events of a certain type take place. For example, electrolyte imbalances and immobility are the conditions under which bed sores develop. The general scientific laws he formulated regarding motion, resistance, and attraction became part of a theory of the universe that existed in the 17th and 18th centuries. Unfortunately, Descartes often used experimentation to help him formulate laws rather than prove their veracity (Losee 2001). He was more of an armchair philosopher than scientist.

Descartes believed that knowledge exists when there are clear and distinct ideas. If an idea is clear and distinct, he reasoned, it must be true. In his method, all ideas are false until, through what he called 'innate knowledge,' it is no longer possible for each idea to be false. This process begins with the statement *cogito ergo sum* – 'I think, therefore I am.' Because a person is aware of his thoughts, he must exist. Descartes posited the existence of a God who created – and gave humans the mind to fathom – everything. Everything that is clear and distinct to the mind is true, as a benevolent God would not mislead humans by giving them a mind that understands things.

Descartes was interested in the epistemology of knowledge, in the ways of knowing. Epistemology, a branch of philosophy, formulates theories about how people acquire a confident knowledge of anything. Descartes' theory of knowledge is based on what one knows, not what one experiences; sensory input is untrustworthy. Instead, one needs to think in an orderly fashion, advancing from the simplest, most easily acquired knowledge to the most complex knowledge. One gains knowledge by breaking things down into smaller and smaller units and rationally reconstructing their order. The goal is to achieve certainty through reflection and reason.

The notion that thought is distinct from the physical body gave rise to the Cartesian mind–body split. Current views about private versus public worlds – that the mind is a private realm, but the body is publicly accessible – stem from this distinction.

Descartes has had an immense influence on Western culture. His ideas stir debate even now. For example, he concluded that because humans are thinking animals, humans are superior. He viewed the world in mechanistic terms, as a conglomeration of small parts interacting directly with each other rather than as an integrated whole. Mind–body dualism has plagued holistic approaches to physical and mental health. Descartes' contention that rational thought is superior to feelings or emotions can cause tension between care providers, who focus only on patients' physical maladies, and patients, who believe the whole self warrants attention.

A countervailing force to rationalism was empiricism, which arose around the same time. The philosophers and scientists in the empiricist group – who were mostly British and included John Locke, Francis Bacon, and David Hume – reacted to Descartes' denigration of sensory experience. In Germany, the empiricist Immanuel Kant tried to meld elements of both viewpoints (Losee 2001). The empiricists' work evolved over time into the scientific realism approach that many nurse scientists use today.

Scientific realism

In the West, science is generally based on empirical observations by people deemed to be experts, and proving or disproving theories is the most accurate and reliable way for researchers to understand phenomena and anticipate events. The ability of science to explain both the observable and the unobservable is a large part of its usefulness in building knowledge (Ladyman 2002). 'Scientific realists' say science can be trusted to describe, with sufficient accuracy, things that cannot be seen.

There are different shades of realism. According to 'direct realists,' much of what humans know about things that exist independently of the mind is based on feedback from one or more of the five senses. However, critics of direct realism argue that sense experience is not independent of the mind at all; rather, because the mind organizes and interprets information through the senses, humans cannot 'directly' comprehend anything without mental processing. The mind's ability to experience, organize, and interpret is implicated in describing things as 'independent,' so to claim that things exist independently of the mind is illogical. Furthermore, they point out that a dreamer 'sees' what appear to be real images, when in fact the mind manufactures them.

'Causal realism' is a modification of direct realism. Its proponents say that if reality begins with information being conveyed to the mind via the senses, then the mind can only perceive things indirectly through the senses (Ladyman 2002). Yet another form of realism is 'idea-ism.' According to this notion, the mind constructs an understanding of the world based not on the inherent qualities of things, but on the way it organizes perceptions into ideas or groups.

In any case, the shift away from direct realism was an important turning point in the history of philosophy because it put an end to naïve claims that people can gain complete knowledge of something outside of their perceptions. John Locke and the other British empiricists successfully promoted the idea that, although things exist apart from the mind, no description of them is possible without primary reference to the mind that perceives them.

The causal realists' and idea-ists' efforts to establish the mind as the center of perception was a giant leap to idealism, promoted by the Irish bishop and philosopher George Berkeley. He said that what people mostly know is their own ideas, so they should speak of things as they perceive them, not of the things themselves.

Kant took a different tack. He maintained that things do exist independently of perception, in the 'nuomenal world,' but that people can only know things in the 'phenomenal world' – what they feel and interpret. This view was a precursor to phenomenologic methods of accruing knowledge. For Locke, humans are a 'blank slate' at birth: They build knowledge over time as sensory experiences are inscribed on the slate. For Kant, humans have *a priori* knowledge derived from pure reason, apart from sensual experience. Mathematical computations are possible, for instance, because of the mind's rational capability, not because of sensory perceptions.

Kant has had a major influence on modern philosophy. He formulated criteria for the acceptability of theories. That is, to be acceptable, theories must have predictive power and testability. He proposed the idea of seeking teleologic explanations for phenomena: Asking questions about 'ends' may suggest new hypotheses about 'means,' which in turn could add to science-based knowledge (Losee 2001). The biologic sciences, in particular, have made useful advances in knowledge by researching the purposes or functions of biologic phenomena.

However, in thinking a little more deeply about science, some people have questioned whether science is of much help in describing things. In 1928, the English physicist Arthur Eddington famously posed a problem concerning the plausibility of scientific descriptions. He illustrated the problem by first citing a commonplace description of a table. It is a solid object with weight, length, breadth, and so on – characteristics all would agree constitute a table. But if a table were then described in terms of atomic theory, as a collection of weightless electrical charges, it consists mostly of emptiness (Ladyman 2002). How does one account for the seemingly vast difference between a table as seen and felt, and what scientific theory would have everyone believe?

One response to this dilemma is to suppose that things have both primary and secondary qualities. 'Primary' qualities are those that seem to coincide with properties of a thing as they are presumed to be scientifically. 'Secondary' refers to qualities as they appear to the mind's eye and that do not coincide with the scientific description. A table's 'bulkiness,' for example, is a secondary quality. But a problem arose regarding secondary qualities. One could argue that qualities such as color, taste, smell, and temperature are not fixed; they can vary depending on the circumstances and the different sensory capabilities of observers. So speaking precisely or meaningfully about secondary qualities can be difficult (Ladyman 2002).

Locke suggested instead that in thinking about how to describe things, one should differentiate between nominal essence (surface appearance) and real essence (what something is in itself), which may be entirely different. For example, a counterfeit $100 bill may appear to be authentic, but in fact is not. According to Locke, scientists who try to perceive real essences of an object are doomed to failure because they can only go as far as their perceptions – what they actually see. It is not possible to reach beyond. However, he also believed that scientists could come to somewhat of a consensus about the accuracy of statements regarding real essences. The unanswered philosophical question is whether an agreed-upon statement is the same as knowing a thing's true nature.

Underlying this question is a more fundamental one: Is it even worthwhile to make claims about real essences apart from the mind that perceives the world?

'Metaphysics' often refers to things beyond the physical, but it also may refer to things beyond perception. Another term for this notion is 'mind-independence.' Scientific realists believe that things exist independently of the mind that perceives them, including things that no one has actually seen but that scientists have described, such as subatomic particles, electrical charges, and orbits (Ladyman 2002).

Twentieth century philosophy of science

In the 1920s, a group of scientists and philosophers met regularly in Vienna to develop 'logical positivism.' They wanted the best, most precise words to accurately describe experiences of things, thus enabling meaningful discussions. Words and concepts such as 'omniscience,' 'God,' and 'things in themselves' that were imprecise and not perceivable through the senses would be excluded and not have a place in meaningful scientific discourse.

According to logical positivists, only science can lead to an understanding of what is true and what is false. They also held that the proper purpose of philosophy is to explain facts related to practical experience rather than concentrating on theory or speculation. They continued their argument by stating that scientific claims of truth are either analytic (using logic to determine meanings and associations of words) or synthetic (using scientific methods to verify assertions). This narrowed the kinds of observations and statements that would qualify as legitimate expressions of scientifically adduced facts. In the end, all language about the world outside of perception was illicit. The only legitimate claims of truth were analytic or based on experiences that many people could confirm under the same observational circumstances.

Much of the logical positivists' work led philosophers to language analysis, or examining how words function to convey meaning. For scientists, this meant accepting the language in concepts or theories as temporary conventions – good enough for the moment and better than any other terms – to explain phenomena. In this view, theories more or less correspond with phenomena, but they are not to be taken literally in the sense that they perfectly describe how unobservable phenomena interact.

In summary, 20th century scientific realists believe that theories can describe phenomena – even unobservable phenomena – that really exist. Moreover, these things exist independently of the mind because the world confirms it and they function in ways that theories can predict and explain. Therefore, the theories are a valid part of knowledge. Most nurses provide patient care based on theories. For example, cardiac output (CO) is described as the relationship between stroke volume (SV) and heart rate (HR). Although nurses cannot see cardiac output, they know it is real and that a theory – $CO = SV \times HR$ – explains it.

Anti-realists, in contrast, may deny or remain uncommitted about things, descriptions of things, or theoretical assertions that are said to be reliable sources of knowledge. Furthermore, theories only reflect a consensus of current opinion among recognized scientists. They point out, for example, that sometimes two or more theories explain the same phenomenon differently. In this situation, some anti-realists say it is appropriate to reserve judgment about which theory, if any, is correct.

Another argument against scientific realism is that, over time, theories change. An example is the once widely held theory of an Earth-centered universe. Because new theories emerge to replace old ones, anti-realists think it is best to embrace current theories lightly, including those that try to accurately describe unobservable things.

Scientific realists reply, with some humility, that at least theories are 'approximately true.' However, this raises a question: What is the difference between something that is only approximately true and something that is simply wrong? A solution may be to shift the force of theory from approximate truth to the serviceability of language used to refer to something. If theoretical language successfully explains and predicts phenomena, realists say, then it is sufficiently valid.

Postmodern philosophy's influence on nursing science

In the late 20th century, philosophers, social scientists, and professionals in the humanities, especially literature, objected to the presumed patriarchal and racist science agendas, which led to major questions regarding the purpose and worthiness of science. Philosophers who studied science from a social perspective attempted to dethrone it from a position of undue and unjustified authority and respect. They said, for example, that stances such as the rejection by scientific leaders of homeopathy as a legitimate health care alternative illustrated a narrow and self-serving posture inconsistent with the best that science claimed about itself. They also denied the epistemic status of other scientific theories (Rosenberg 2000).

An upheaval in the social sciences, and to a lesser extent the basic sciences, occurred in the 1970s and 1980s. Researchers who favored qualitative methods argued that those who used quantitative methods were simply aping physical scientists and that this approach would not lead to an understanding of many human problems. The divide between qualitative and quantitative paradigms in the social sciences has become a major area of interest for philosophers of science – in particular, whether quantitative methods for seeking objective truth should be abandoned.

Postmodern philosophy rejects the notion of a single reality – that there is only one way to obtain truth – and the 'meta-narratives' warranting this interpretation. It maintains that multiple cultural, social, economic, and other factors influence knowledge claims, and that multiple interpretations and less obvious meanings are important in understanding the 'margins' of such claims (Rodgers 2005). These tenets run counter to key presuppositions upon which, for more than 2000 years, scientists and philosophers of science had based their quest for knowledge. Indeed, postmodernism is an entirely different approach to the development of knowledge, one that does not depend on Francis Bacon's scientific method or designing a 'perfect theory' to explain everything in nature. It relies instead on qualitative methods.

Postmodern philosophy arose in parallel to the thinking of Thomas Kuhn, Larry Laudan, and Stephen Toulmin – historicists who believed that knowledge of history is the only way to gain a true understanding of the world. Historicism was a thoughtful reaction to the legacy of authoritarianism, racism, colonialism, sexism, and heterosexism. Postmodern historicists critically examine value statements about the origins of knowledge, creating a new 'world view' (Rosenberg 2000). This world view, in turn, has led to the development of critical social theory, feminist theory, and various forms of deconstruction.

Feminist philosophy has been important to nurse scientists because many of the phenomena they study are similar to those examined by social scientists. For example, instead of simply accepting the medico-centric approach to, and the meta-narratives surrounding, labor and delivery in childbirth, nurse researchers have sought to understand the unique perspectives of women by gathering qualitative data from them. The findings from such studies have improved women's childbirth experiences. Similarly, in studying the unique experiences of women after myocardial infarction or cardiac surgery, researchers have taken into account multiple cultural, social, economic, gender, and other factors.

The postmodernist tenet that multiple interpretations and less obvious meanings are important in understanding the 'margins' may also apply to the disability, pain, and other travails that people experience daily. While such experiences may not be of primary concern to the medical community, they are of interest to nurse scientists. Those who study symptoms of illness – for example, constipation in elderly women – have shed new light on the meaning of these phenomena.

Postmodernists recognize the importance and power of language in shaping thoughts, behavior, and action. Science, they maintain, is privileged in the sense that relatively few people understand its language (Rodgers 2005). Some feminist philosophers argue that this puts women at a disadvantage because the domination of science by men privileges their work over the work of women, who frequently have not had easy access to scientific language or laboratories.

In the 1980s and 1990s, nurse researchers and others in the social sciences and humanities often engaged in heated debate about quantitative versus qualitative methods. As the discipline of nursing matured and scholars were thoroughly exposed to a variety of methods, the heat became a low simmer. Today, the two camps acknowledge that gains in nursing knowledge require both quantitative and qualitative approaches. Equally important, they realize that research questions and the methods used to answer them must be aligned – that ideology should not drive methodology.

Conclusions

Philosophers since the early Greeks have had an influence on nursing science. Over the centuries, they have grappled with core issues such as the role of quantitative versus qualitative analysis in efforts to advance knowledge. Nursing, like other disciplines, has had to come to terms with these different methods. Today, it acknowledges that both approaches can contribute to knowledge development.

Although the philosophy of nursing science is still in its infancy compared to most other sciences, nursing's growth and successful preparation of well-qualified researchers in the last 20 years have placed the discipline in an enviable position. It has achieved recognition by the National Institutes of Health (NIH) in the USA and by similar entities elsewhere, such as the Canadian Institute of Health Research. Nurse scientists compete well for research funds from all NIH institutes, and their work is recognized in highly respected health science and social science journals.

These and other accomplishments make nursing science well-prepared for the philosophical debates ahead.

References

Fawcett, J. (1984) The metaparadigm of nursing: Current status and future refinements. *Journal of Nursing Scholarship*, **16**(3), 84–87.

Holmes, D. & Gastaldo, D. (2004) Rhizomatic thought in nursing: An alternative path for the development of the discipline. *Nursing Philosophy*, **5**(3), 258–267.

Ladyman, J. (2002) *Understanding philosophy of science*. New York: Routledge Press.

Losee, J. (2001) *A historical introduction to the philosophy of science*, 4th Edn. Oxford: Oxford University Press.

Rodgers, B. (2005) *Developing nursing knowledge: Philosophical traditions and influences.* Philadelphia: Lippincott Williams & Wilkins.

Rosenberg, A. (2000) *Philosophy of science: A contemporary introduction.* New York: Routledge Press.

Chapter 3
Theory and nursing science

Carmen J. Portillo & William L. Holzemer

Introduction

Theory development in nursing has not been a magical process, but rather a systematic one that has evolved rapidly in the last four decades (Alligood 2002). Florence Nightingale (1992) pioneered the systematic collection of observations, actions, and perceptions of nursing in the 19th century to produce the first concept of nursing. In her early edicts, she wrote that nurses use a knowledge base that is different from the knowledge base physicians use. However, the nursing profession did not begin discussing the need to develop, articulate, and test nursing theory until about 100 years later.

Modern nursing theory began in the 1960s with the likes of Virginia Henderson. In her grand theory of nursing, Henderson defined nursing as 'assisting individuals to gain independence in the performance of activities contributing to health or its recovery' (Henderson 1966, p. 15). Theory development has since evolved into four general kinds of theoretical works (Alligood 2002). This chapter focuses on three of them: grand, middle-range, and situation-specific theories.

Types of theory

Grand theories are broad in scope and often emphasize relationships that are difficult to test. In addition to Henderson's grand theory, examples include Martha Rogers' science of unitary human being, Margaret Newman's health and expanding consciousness, and Rosemarie Parse's theory of human becoming.

Middle-range theories are more modest in scope, more precise, and focused on answering specific nursing questions; they potentially can be validated through research. Examples are Cheryl Tatano Beck's postpartum depression theory, Ramona Mercer's maternal role attainment theory, and Merle Mishel's uncertainty in illness theory.

Table 3.1 Theoretical levels and adherents.

Level	Adherents
Grand Systematic constructions of the nature and mission of nursing, and of nursing care goals, based on a synthesis of experiences, observations, insights, and research findings	Henderson (1966) King (1971, 1995, 1997) Levine (1973, 1991) Newman (1986) Orem (1971) Parse (1981) Rogers (1970, 1983, 1986)
Middle-range Narrowly focused, more concrete than grand theories. Address specific phenomena or concepts, and reflect nursing practice	Beck (2002a, 2002b) Mercer (1977, 1986, 1995) Mishel (1981, 1990) Reed (1991) Reed & Shearer (2004)
Situation-specific Focused on specific nursing phenomena that reflect clinical practice. Usually limited to specific populations or to a particular field of practice. Research scope and questions also are limited and encompass a specific context, such as HIV/AIDS prevention in African-American adolescents (Jemmott & Jemmott 2000), stigma (Holzemer et al. 2007), and pain (Melzack & Wall 1965)	Holzemer et al. (2007) Jemmott & Jemmott (2000) Jemmott et al. (2001) Melzack & Wall (1965)

Today, many nurse researchers use situation-specific theories, which are more closely linked to clinical practice. Table 3.1 summarizes these three levels of theory and cites some of their adherents.

Educators have spent a great deal of energy moving middle-range theories into academic curricula. However, it has been very difficult moving from theory-based nursing education to applying a middle-range theory such as self-care in clinical practice. There seems to be less need today for nursing to have its 'own' theory describing how people live, adapt, become ill, recover, and heal. Rather, nursing science uses physiologic processes and cognitive behavioral theories to attempt to understand individuals, families, and communities and how they experience their health, illness, and wellness.

The profession is excited about, and focusing energy on, evidence-based practice and practice-based evidence to build knowledge about effective delivery of care. Often, evidence-based practice represents a quantitative perspective, and practice-based evidence a qualitative perspective, on building knowledge. Sometimes they also represent, respectively, deductive and inductive perspectives. Although the randomized controlled trial is the gold standard for research in building evidence-based practice, there is growing awareness of the method's limitations and related ethical dilemmas, such as giving a placebo to the control group. Practice-based evidence suggests a need for electronic information systems to capture the assessments, interventions, and outcomes of interest to nursing practice so data mining can occur, yet few health care environments are currently able to build such evidence empirically. However, there are efforts to capture practice-based evidence through interpretative research methods.

Recently, the Western Pacific and South-East Asia regions of the World Health Organization formally adopted a new theoretical model of people-centered care comprising four domains: informed and empowered individuals, families, and communities; competent and responsive health practitioners; efficient and benevolent health care organizations; and supportive and humanitarian health care systems (World Health Organization 2007). People-centered care is a paradigm shift away from today's health care system, which is too biomedically oriented, disease-focused, technology-driven, and doctor-dominated.

People-centered care is a vision of health care that harmonizes the mind and body, people, and systems and seeks to re-establish the health and well-being of people as the central goal. It is a rich and complex vision with the potential to guide nursing practice as a significant component of a humanized, interdisciplinary health system (Holzemer 2008).

Components of theory

Authors have articulated various components of theory. Hage (1972), a sociologist, and nursing researchers Dulock and Holzemer (1991) wrote about concepts and constructs, and how these are related through theoretical and operational systems. For example, theoretical systems provide statements about the relationship between pain and quality of life. Dulock and Holzemer (1991) used the term substruction to describe a strategy for thinking about how theory and research are linked.[1]

Concepts and constructs are the building blocks of theory. Statements about the relationships between them describe how variables are related. A concept is an abstract or concrete mental image of a phenomenon; it can be graded in terms of the level of abstraction. More general and abstract concepts are often referred to as constructs. Statements about the relationships between concepts and constructs become an ontology – a formal representation of concepts within a domain. For example, early authors wrote that the domain of nursing comprises four constructs: person, environment, health and illness, and nursing (Yura & Torres 1975). According to this definition, nursing care focuses on the person's health and illness in the context of his or her environment. These constructs are broad and not very helpful from a research perspective, but they draw boundaries around how to think about nursing and patients, families, and community care.

The literature on theory can be confusing because authors ascribe different meanings to some terms. 'Paradigm,' 'framework,' 'model,' and 'theory' often are used interchangeably. In this chapter, theory means a statement about concepts and constructs that provides a basis for examining the potential relationships between them. For example, pain is a construct that may include three related concepts – pain intensity, location, and duration; quality of life is a construct that may include the concepts of physical, mental, and social health. A theory might relate pain and quality of life by suggesting that the greater the pain, the worse the quality of life. More specifically, one might theorize that pain intensity is more closely related to physical health than mental health.

A theory is a statement of knowledge about a topic based on the available evidence. For example, evidence supports the notion that turning patients frequently and keeping them in a dry bed reduces the risk of skin breakdown. The theory addresses patients at risk for skin breakdown in the context of an environment where there is a specific illness condition, and also addresses the potential for a nursing intervention. Nursing theory is different from other kinds of theory in that it focuses on nursing actions or interventions. Many non-nursing theorists are not concerned about patient care or actions/interventions.

By deductive or inductive means, nurse scientists build knowledge or theory for nursing practice, as described in Chapter 2. Theoretical relationships among constructs can be tested deductively, or knowledge embedded in practice can be built inductively. These two creative processes are significant for both the discipline and profession of nursing. Theoretical development provides a cohesive, systematic view of theoretical knowledge and its application to practice. At one time, nursing focused solely on knowledge about how nurses function. Today, theoretical development focuses on what nurses know and how they use that knowledge to guide their training, decision-making, and care.

Authors have articulated strategies for evaluating nursing-related knowledge or theories. Walker and Avant (2005) proposed that, in analyzing a theory, one should understand how it developed or the data that support it, understand how the constructs and concepts are related, assess the usefulness of information the theory yields, and determine its applicability to other conditions, its parsimony (simplicity), and its testability. Meleis (2007) discussed the relationship between and among constructs and concepts using the terms 'clarity,' 'consistency,' 'simplicity,' and 'tautology.' Tautology refers to circularity in a theoretical argument – for example, patients' quality of life affects their post-hospitalization quality of life. Circularity in theoretical knowledge is not very helpful.

Nursing definitions and theory

One way to understand nursing theory better is to examine several definitions of nursing itself, then ask, 'What is the theory behind these definitions?' Do they shed light on the concepts and constructs of interest to nursing and how they might be related? Here are three online definitions:

(1) International Council of Nurses: 'Nursing encompasses autonomous and collaborative care of individuals of all ages, families, groups, and communities, sick or well, and in all settings. Nursing includes the promotion of health, prevention of illness, and the care of ill, disabled and dying people.'
(2) Japan Nurses Association: 'Nursing is defined as to assist the individual and the group, sick or well, to maintain, promote and restore health.'
(3) American Nurses Association: 'Nursing is the assessment, diagnose, and treatment of human responses.'

In this exercise, it is helpful to recall the four domains identified by Yura and Torres (1975): person (individual, family, and community); health (wellness, and acute and chronic illness); environment (across settings); and nursing (care, interventions, and treatments). Are all the domains represented in the three nursing definitions? These domains can be used to organize the constructs and concepts implied by theory.

Theory enables researchers to identify the variables they want to study. Linking theory to research methods makes it possible to describe the dimensions of the four domains by exploring the potential relationships among constructs and concepts. The ultimate goal of linking theory with research is to explain or predict relationships among the domains.

Conclusions

Theory is at the core of science. It provides a framework for thinking about phenomena and research methods, and for disseminating findings to clinical practice.

Nursing has a rich history of developing scholarship, beginning with Florence Nightingale's environmental theory. She defined environment as 'all the external conditions and influences affecting the life and development of an organism and capable of preventing, suppressing, or contributing to disease, accidents, or death' (Murray & Zentner 1975, p. 149). If nursing science is to advance and provide evidence for practice, thus enabling clinicians to influence patient care positively, scholars must continue developing, adapting, and adopting theories. This requires collaboration with other researchers, clinical practitioners, and health professionals in other fields. Physiologic and cognitive behavioral theories are guiding much of today's research on patient care. Nurse scientists can have a significant role in that effort.

Note

1   A strategy for how to think about theory and research, called the Outcomes Model for Health Care Research, is described in Chapters 7 and 12.

References

Alligood, M.R. (2002) Models and theories in nursing practice. In M.R. Alligood & A.M. Tomey (Eds) *Nursing theory: Utilization and application*, 2nd Edn. (pp. 3–14). St. Louis, MO: Mosby.

Beck, C.T. (2002a) A meta-synthesis of qualitative research. *American Journal of Maternal Child Nursing* **27**(4), 214–221.

Beck, C.T. (2002b) Revision of the postpartum depression predictors inventory. *Journal of Obstetric, Gynecologic, & Neonatal Nursing* **31**(4), 394–402.

Dulock, H. & Holzemer, W.L. (1991) Substruction: Improving the linkage from theory to method. *Nursing Science Quarterly* **4**(2), 83–87.

Hage, J. (1972) *Techniques and problems of theory construction in sociology*. New York: John Wiley & Sons.

Henderson, V. (1966) *The nature of nursing*. New York: Macmillan.

Holzemer, W.L. (2008) Nursing theory: Remembering our future. *Japanese Journal of Nursing Research* **5**(2), 71.

Holzemer, W.L., Uys, L., Makoae, L., Stewart, A., Phetlhu, R., Dlamini, P., et al. (2007) A conceptual model of HIV/AIDS stigma from five African countries. *Journal of Advanced Nursing* **58**(6), 541–551.

Jemmott, J.B. III & Jemmott, L.S. (2000) HIV risk reduction behavioral interventions with heterosexual adolescents. *AIDS* **14**(Suppl 2), S40–S52.

Jemmott, J.B. III, Jemmott, L.S., Hines, P.M. & Fong, G.T. (2001) The theory of planned behavior as a model of intentions for fighting among African American and Latino adolescents. *Maternal Child Health* **5**(4), 253–263.

King, I.M. (1971) *Toward a theory for nursing: General concepts of human behavior.* New York: John Wiley & Sons.

King, I.M. (1995) A systems framework for nursing. In M.A. Frey & C.L. Sieloff (Eds) *Advancing King's systems framework and theory of nursing* (pp. 14–32). Thousand Oaks, CA: Sage.

King, I.M. (1997) Reflections on the past and a vision for the future. *Nursing Science Quarterly* **10**(1), 15–17.

Levine, M.E. (1973) *Introduction to clinical nursing*, 2nd Edn. Philadelphia: F.A. Davis.

Levine, M.E. (1991) The conservation principles: A model for health. In K. Schaefer & J. Pond (Eds) *Levine's Conservation Model: A framework for nursing practice* (pp. 1–11). Philadelphia: F.A. Davis.

Meleis, A.I. (2007) *Theoretical nursing: Development and progress*, 4th Edn. Philadelphia: Lippincott Williams & Wilkins.

Melzack, R. & Wall, P.D. (1965) Pain mechanisms: A new theory. *Science* **150**, 971–979.

Mercer, R.T. (1977) *Nursing care for parents at risk*. Thorofare, NJ: Charles B. Slack.

Mercer, R.T. (1986) *First-time motherhood: Experiences from teens to forties.* New York: Springer.

Mercer, R.T. (1995) *Becoming a mother: Research on maternal identity from Rubin to the present.* New York: Springer.

Mishel, M.H. (1981) The measurement of uncertainty in illness. *Nursing Research* **30**(5), 258–263.

Mishel, M.H. (1990) Reconceptualization of the uncertainty in illness theory. *Journal of Nursing Scholarship* **22**(4), 256–262.

Murray, R. & Zentner, J. (1975) *Nursing concepts in health promotion*. Englewood Cliffs, NJ: Prentice Hall.

Newman, M. (1986) *Health as expanding consciousness*. St. Louis, MO: C.V. Mosby.

Nightingale, F. (1992) *Notes on nursing: What it is, and what it is not*, Commemorative Edition. London: Lippincott Williams & Wilkins.

Orem, D.E. (1971) *Nursing: Concepts of practice*. New York: McGraw-Hill.

Parse, R.R. (1981) *Man-living-health: A theory of nursing*. New York: John Wiley & Sons.

Reed, P.G. (1991) Toward a nursing theory of self-transcendence: Deductive reformulation using developmental theories. *Advances in Nursing Science* **13**(4), 64–77.

Reed, P.G. & Shearer, N. (Eds). (2004) *Perspectives on nursing theory*, 4th Edn. New York: Lippincott Williams & Wilkins.

Rogers, M.E. (1970) *An introduction to the theoretical basis of nursing*. Philadelphia: F.A. Davis.

Rogers, M.E. (1983) Science of unitary human beings: A paradigm for nursing. In I.W. Clements & F.B. Roberts (Eds) *Family health: A theoretical approach to nursing care* (pp. 219–227). New York: John Wiley & Sons.

Rogers, M.E. (1986) Science of unitary human beings. In V.M. Malinski (Ed) *Explorations in Martha Rogers' science of unitary human beings* (pp. 3–8). Norwalk, CT: Appleton-Century-Crofts.

Walker, L. & Avant, K. (2005) *Strategies for theory construction in nursing*, 4th Edn. Upper Saddle River, NJ: Pearson Prentice Hall.

World Health Organization, South-East Asia Region and Western Pacific Region (2007) *People at the centre of health care: Harmonizing mind and body, people and systems.* Geneva: WHO.

Yura, H. & Torres, G. (1975) *Today's conceptual framework with baccalaureate nursing programs.* Publication No. 15-1558, 17-75. New York: National League for Nursing.

Part 2
Nursing research: making a difference in people's lives

Chapter 4
Improving patient care

Suzanne Willard

Introduction

Nurses are present at the most intimate times in peoples' lives. They provide quality care – the essence of nursing – based on findings by nurse scientists, whose recommendations regarding interventions have an impact on care. In this sense, researchers and clinicians work together to ensure the best clinical outcomes.

This chapter reviews some of the innovative research that has improved patient care and outcomes.

Nursing research and clinical practice

Research by nurses provides a foundation for clinical practice. Whether nurses are researchers, educators, or clinicians, it is important that they disseminate and use research findings because patients benefit from new knowledge. Today's communication technologies make it easier than ever for the global nursing community to share research findings and much more. Via the Internet, nurses around the world can quickly access important information and integrate research findings into patient care.

In looking at nursing from a global perspective, Montgomery et al. (2001) recommended seven ways to foster nursing research and the application of findings:

(1) Integrate research methods and uses into educational curricula at all levels;
(2) Encourage educational institutions to collaborate creatively;
(3) Use international nursing research conferences as a means to disseminate more information about research activities;
(4) Make the dissemination and use of research findings a priority in clinical settings;
(5) Establish and support an international committee to coordinate research dissemination efforts;

(6)   Use creative efforts and funding to enhance access to research findings; and
(7)   Make research publications more reader-friendly for practicing nurses.

The intersection of nursing science and nursing practice has important implications for health care worldwide. Cross-border cooperation and information exchange provide a global view of prevalent health problems and inform nurse researchers about everyday nursing issues that need to be addressed. International collaborations such as the University of California, San Francisco (UCSF) Nursing HIV/AIDS Center[1] enable nurses to share knowledge about common themes, including symptom management, disease prevention, end-of-life care, and pain management. The World Health Organization and the International Council of Nurses also promote collaboration to foster research on widespread nursing challenges.

Symptom management

A challenge for nurses globally is developing disease-specific symptom management strategies. Managing symptoms that patients experience during illness, based on how they perceive it, has been a core value of the nursing profession. Each patient's experience with a disease is unique as he or she responds to physical changes and to changes in thoughts or cognition of the response. There may be a cluster of symptoms indicative of multiple diseases. For example, increased thirst may indicate diabetes or one of many other diseases, and headache could be associated with migraine or a sinus infection. The distress a patient feels is frequently the most relevant factor affecting his or her symptomatic response. Patients with a poor quality of life and low adherence to the necessary medication regimen often report a high rate of symptoms.

Symptoms can deter improved clinical outcomes in HIV disease, a lifelong chronic illness. To improve the outcomes of people living with HIV, Sprig et al. (2005) recommended that clinical nurses and researchers collaborate to understand patients' symptom experiences and social systems. Their review of the literature revealed a poor understanding among patients of the impact of HIV symptoms, and they strongly recommended that nurses focus on building relationships with, and support networks for, patients. Evidence-based guidelines for symptom management have been outlined (Holzemer 2002).

Miles et al. (2003), who have worked with low-income African-American women, studied another approach to managing the symptoms of HIV: a cognitive reframing protocol that provided information about the disease and self-care symptom management. Such women, they found, delay seeking medical care and present with advanced disease. The researchers applied the protocol in women's homes in an effort to overcome the stigma that often is associated with an HIV diagnosis and that can stifle participation in such a study. Based on their literature review, the researchers knew that women with HIV disease also have a high level of depression, which has been correlated with an increase in symptoms. The best interventions, this study showed, were those that addressed the social context of the disease – specifically, the related mental health issues and depressive symptoms.

Symptoms also have an adverse effect on adherence to medications, research suggests. Holzemer et al. (1999) studied the relationships between the five dimensions of the Wilson and Cleary model of health-related quality of life – biological and physiological factors, symptoms, functioning, general health perceptions, and overall quality of life – and three self-reported adherence measures in persons living with HIV. They found that HIV-infected individuals who had elevated symptom scores, particularly for depression, were more likely not to adhere to their medication regimes, not to follow the advice of their health care provider, and to miss more appointments. Conversely, participants who reported having a meaningful life and felt well cared for were more likely to take their medications and heed their health care provider's advice.

Clinical pathways have received attention because they provide a road map to nursing care problems. Olsson et al. (2007) used a pathway for patients with hip fracture, taking an integrated care approach that involved a multidisciplinary team of nurses, physicians, and physical therapists. Their quasi-experimental prospective study assessed the motivation of patients (excluding those whose hip fracture was pathologic and those with severe dementia) to return to optimum health, by measuring and analyzing qualitative data. Twenty-one percent of patients in the intervention group were restored to their pre-fracture quality of life, compared to only 5% in the comparison group. The researchers recommended an intensive, holistic assessment upon admission, ensuring a plan of care that would meet the patient's needs. The study results led to a best practice statement for managing hip fracture patients and related symptoms that became part of routine care at the institution where the research took place.

In another study, Campbell (2006) demonstrated the effectiveness of a multidisciplinary team in caring for all infants. Care included interventions, parent education, and recommendations for follow-up after discharge. The author concluded that team members were able to ensure safe, consistent, quality care. According to Campbell, clinical pathways can improve care and organize it. In the neonatal field, it is crucial that evidence-based guidelines are tailored to specific populations (Campbell 2006).

Chronic obstructive pulmonary disease (COPD) poses many challenges to nursing. In addition to understanding the physiologic aspects of this disease, nurses need to be aware that it can cause intense anxiety in patients as they struggle to breathe. A study of COPD patients by Lee et al. (2002) assessed the impact of a care protocol that nurses in China designed for community nurses to use in collaboration with nursing home staff. The researchers measured functional, respiratory, and psychologic data for patients who received either the care protocol or no intervention. They also looked at hospital service utilization, different types of nursing home staff (based on their level of education), and patient satisfaction. While there was no difference between the two groups in terms of functional or respiratory outcomes, or service utilization, there was significant improvement in psychologic well-being among patients who underwent the care protocol. Well-being is an important factor for chronically ill people, yet health care workers often get lost in attending to physiologic aspects. The researchers found that using community nurses gave patients the support they needed to cope with COPD.

Ervin et al. (2004), working with heart failure patients in the home using a model of care that links academic-nursing and clinical-nursing services, noted improved outcomes with an evidenced-based protocol. They also studied the implementation of this evidence-based nursing care protocol to enhance patients' quality of life. In abstracting data from patient charts (charting has a key role in continuity of care) before this protocol was in place, the researchers found incongruous documentation of patient education. After it was implemented, documentation improved, enabling consistent care. The protocol cued staff about specific aspects of teaching and about patients' assessment needs. Importantly, the authors concluded that integrating research findings into front-line nursing practice often does not occur.

Nurses who are beginning their career can easily become immersed in the day-to-day demands of clinical work. In designing the Nursing Research Internship Program, which gives practicing nurses an opportunity to grow professionally, Wells et al. (2007) sought to overcome perceived barriers to evidence-based practice. They found that nurses who participated in the program learned to use scientific literature not only to solve clinical problems, but also to identify problems that may not have been evident. This framework, to which the participants may not have been exposed in their primary nursing education, will guide their lifelong quest for knowledge.

Disease prevention

There are many opportunities for nurses to deliver prevention messages in their daily work. However, educational initiatives must be tailored to patients' particular needs and level of understanding. Coleman and Ball (2007) studied perceived barriers to condom use during sexual encounters among HIV-infected men who were African-American, middle aged or older, and living in the USA. The biggest barriers to condom use in this group were having fewer symptoms and being single. The researchers concluded that in order to increase condom use, HIV prevention efforts in the USA and abroad should be customized for this particular population.

Disclosure of a person's HIV diagnosis to others also may have an impact on how the individual responds to treatment recommendations. Bairan et al. (2007) developed a disclosure model, based on the type of social relationships among study participants, that nurses and other health care providers could use in routine clinical encounters. For the purpose of data analysis, the researchers characterized these relationships as either sexual or non-sexual, then correlated the depth of a relationship with the ability to disclose the diagnosis. Disclosure turned out to be a complex phenomenon. Even when treatment is good, HIV still brings great fear and stigma to social relationships.

HIV prevention among adolescents in poor African countries where vast numbers of HIV-infected people live is urgently needed. Chrissie Kaponda, a nurse scientist in Malawi, along with colleagues there and at the University of Illinois developed a pilot HIV-prevention program targeted to adolescents. The program was based on risky youth behaviors they observed and on community, cultural, contextual, and other factors that shape them. Incorporating lessons learned from the research and, importantly, gaining buy-in from adolescents and the community contributed to the program's success (Kaponda et al. 2007).

Other HIV-prevention researchers have identified common group themes. Lesser et al. (2007) reported that people in the USA who suffered abuse as children had a high rate of risky behaviors. They designed an intervention to ensure that abuse-related issues would be addressed among adolescents who were pregnant and/or a parent. This unique group of people demonstrated that young parenthood gives them a hope for a better future. The researchers concluded that the abuse component of their intervention was intrinsic to the success of reaching these adolescents, motivating behavioral change, and promoting a sense of resiliency to achieve life success.

Nurse researchers have also devoted a great deal of attention to health promotion and preventing other diseases. In Norway, for example, Tonstad et al. (2007) looked at whether counseling by nurses had an effect on risk factors in patients with hypertension. Although counseling did not reduce blood pressure, it did reduce some of the metabolic risk factors associated with poorly controlled hypertension.

End-of-life care

Having nurses provide end-of-life care was a goal even in the early days of the hospice movement. In an ethnographic study, Wright (2002) identified and described the qualities of nurses who work in this environment. Among the 12 themes that emerged, the most prominent quality was attending to, or being humanly present with, the patient.

End-of-life care also involves giving support to the families of terminally ill patients. Phipps et al. (2003) found that family members caring for such a patient could identify someone outside the immediate family who was helping them. Nevertheless, these family members experienced substantial emotional and financial difficulties. Nurses working in hospices need to understand that even if caregivers in the home have support, they do not take full advantage of resources available to them.

There are mental health consequences for caregivers tending a relative who has dementia, according to Brereton and Nolan (2000). Their study, which also identified some of the ways that families cope with the stress of caregiving, found that 68% of caregivers were highly burdened and 65% exhibited depressive symptoms. The researchers concluded that nurses need to train caregivers individually, especially women, in how to understand and manage the behavior of relatives with dementia, and how to cope with their own emotions. Furthermore, nurses must recognize that caregivers' needs change over time and must learn how to provide the most effective support.

Pain management

A major challenge for the nursing profession is effective pain management, a potentially rich subject for nurse researchers. In a pilot study, Barnason et al. (1998) used a self-study educational program and a structured intervention to improve nurses' critical thinking in managing pain. A structured intervention is consistent and reproducible regardless of who is providing it. Outcomes showed that nurses' knowledge about pain management increased significantly, patient satisfaction improved, and institutional nursing programs focusing on better pain management are key. Because all of the participants received consistent training, pain management was consistent.

Clinical nurse specialists led the intervention in this study. They became a resource for further education of nursing staff about pain management, which improved staff's ability to collaborate supportively in making clinical decisions regarding individual patients. The researchers also noted the pivotal role of the clinical nurse specialist in keeping the pain management protocol consistent, and the importance of emphasizing the positive rather than the negative aspects of patient outcomes.

Pain can produce anxiety and anxiety can produce pain, a cycle that is often difficult to break. Kemppainen et al. (2006), who studied an international HIV-positive population, offered solutions for reducing anxiety. They found that complementary and/or alternative therapies, including prayer, meditation, and relaxation techniques, were the most effective. Patients who attended support groups and exercised also experienced less anxiety. Watching television and talking with family and friends were the most frequently reported strategies. As patients with HIV learn to live with this potentially devastating disease, nurses should help them identify and use methods that patients themselves think are important, the researchers recommended.

The impact of spirituality and religion on pain has received little research attention, although nurses have long acknowledged the intersection of spirituality and health. After a literature review, Unruh (2007), a Canadian nurse, concluded that respectful communication with patients about their pain experiences and the role of spirituality and religion in coping with pain are important. Bedard et al. (2006) employed a multidisciplinary pain management program to demonstrate that effective pain management reduces hospital stays, postoperative complications, and costs.

At a care facility in Jordan, Abushaikha et al. (2005) studied 100 patients who delivered vaginally in a hospital. All of the patients reported that their labor was painful and that they did not receive pain-relief interventions. This finding prompted the facility to adopt new pain-relief measures and alter nurses' role in alleviating pain during labor.

Conclusions

Nursing strategies to improve patient care – including those highlighted in this chapter, which are applicable in all practice settings – have demonstrated a positive impact. Nurses are critical thinkers who use problem-solving skills to help patients and their family caregivers. When nurse scientists and clinicians work together, patient outcomes improve. For the benefit of patients, it is imperative that health professionals share knowledge.

References

Abushaikha, L. & Oweis, A. (2005) Labour pain experience and intensity: A Jordanian perspective. *International Journal of Nursing Practice* **11**(1), 33–38.

Bairan, A., Taylor, G.A., Blake, B.J., Akers, T., Sowell, R. & Mendiola R. Jr. (2007) A model of HIV disclosure: Disclosure and types of social relationships. *Journal of the American Academy of Nurse Practitioners* **19**(5), 242–250.

Barnason, S., Merboth, M., Pozehl, B. & Tietjen, M.J. (1998) Utilizing an outcomes approach to improve pain management by nurses: A pilot study. *Clinical Nurse Specialist* **12**(1), 28–36.

Bedard, D., Purden, M., Sauve-Larose, N., Certosini, C. & Schein, C. (2006) The pain experience of post surgical patients following the implementation of an evidence-based approach. *Pain Management Nursing* **7**(3), 80–92.

Brereton, L. & Nolan, M. (2000) 'You do know he's had a stroke, don't you?' Preparation for family care-giving: The neglected dimension. *Journal of Clinical Nursing* **9**(4), 498–506.

Campbell, M. (2006) Development of a clinical pathway for near term and convalescing premature infants in a level II nursery. *Advances in Neonatal Care* **6**(3), 150–164.

Coleman, C.L. & Ball, K. (2007) Determinants of perceived barriers to condom use among HIV-infected middle-aged and older African-American men. *Journal of Advanced Nursing* **60**(4), 368–376.

Ervin, N., Scrivener, K. & Simons, T. (2004) Using the linkage model for integrating evidence into home care nursing practice. *Home Healthcare Nurse* **22**(9), 606–611.

Holzemer, W.L. (2002) HIV and AIDS: The symptom experience. What cell counts and viral loads won't tell you? *American Journal of Nursing* **102**(4), 48–52.

Holzemer, W.L., Corless, I.B., Nokes, K.M., Turner, J.G., Brown, M.A., Powell-Cope, G.M., et al. (1999) Predictors of self-reported adherence in persons living with HIV disease. *AIDS Patient Care and STDs* **13**(3), 185–197.

Kaponda, C.P., Dancy, B.L., Norr, K.F., Kachingwe, S.I., Mbeba, M.M. & Jere, D.L. (2007) Research brief: Community consultation to develop an acceptable and effective adolescent HIV prevention intervention. *Journal of the Association of Nurses in AIDS Care* **18**(2), 72–77.

Kemppainen, J.K., Eller, L.S., Bunch, E., Hamilton, M.J., Dole, P., Holzemer, W., et al. (2006) Strategies for self-management of HIV-related anxiety. *AIDS Care* **18**(6), 597–607.

Lee, D., Lee, I.F.K., Mackenzie, A. & Ho, R.N.L. (2002) Effects of a care protocol on care outcomes in older nursing home patients with chronic obstructive pulmonary disease. *Journal of the American Geriatric Society* **50**(5), 870–876.

Lesser, J., Koniak-Griffin, D., Gonzalez-Figueroa, E., Huang, R. & Cumberland, W.G. (2007) Childhood abuse history and risk behaviors among teen parents in a culturally rooted, couple-focused HIV prevention program. *Journal of the Association of Nurses in AIDS Care* **18**(2):18–27.

Miles, M., Holditch-Davis, D., Eron, J., Black, B., Pedersen, C. & Harris, D. (2003) An HIV self-care symptom management intervention for African-American mothers. *Nursing Research* **52**(6), 350–360.

Montgomery, K., Eddy, N., Jackson, E., Nelson, E., Reed, K., Stark, T., et al. (2001) Global research dissemination and utilization: Recommendations for nurses and nurse educators. *Nursing & Health Care Perspectives* **22**(3), 124–129.

Olsson, L., Karlsson, J. & Ekman, I. (2007) Effects of nursing interventions within an integrated care pathway for patients with hip fracture. *Journal of Advanced Nursing* **58**(2), 116–125.

Phipps, E., Braitman, L.E., True, G., Harris, D. & Tester, W. (2003) Family care giving for patients at life's end: Report from the cultural variations study (CVAS). *Palliative & Supportive Care* **1**(2), 165–170.

Sprig, R., Moody, K., Battegay, M. & De Geest, S. (2005) Symptom management in HIV/AIDS: Advancing the conceptualization. *Advances in Nursing Science* **28**(4), 333–344.

Tonstad, S., Alm, C. & Sandvik, E. (2007) Effect of nurse counseling on metabolic risk factors in patients with mild hypertension: A randomized controlled trial. *European Journal of Cardiovascular Nursing* **6**(2), 160–164.

Unruh, A.M. (2007) Spirituality, religion, and pain. *Canadian Journal of Nursing Research* **39**(2), 66–86.

Wells, N., Free, M. & Adam, R. (2007) Nursing research internship: Enhancing evidence-based practice among staff nurses. *Journal of Administration* **37**(3), 135–143.

Wright, D. (2002) Researching the qualities of hospice nurses. *Journal of Hospice & Palliative Nursing* **4**(4), 210–216.

Chapter 5
Enhancing care delivery

Mary A. Blegen & Julaluk Baramee

Introduction

More potential exists today than at any time in history for human survival and good health throughout life. More infants survive, more adults live longer, and an increasing number of diseases can be controlled or even eliminated. Yet many people cannot expect to benefit from these health care improvements because the delivery of care is so uneven, creating a moral crisis. Great disparities in health roughly parallel the large and ever-widening disparities in income. How can nurses and nurse researchers address the health-related disparities and create care delivery methods to reduce them?

Nurses constitute the largest group of health care providers worldwide (World Health Organization 2006a). They contribute to health in many delivery venues – acute emergency care (including disasters), inpatient hospital care, chronic long-term care, community primary care, prevention of communicable diseases, health promotion, and community education. This chapter identifies key issues regarding health care delivery by nurses that warrant more research, grouped into five categories: the supply of nurses, measuring nursing care, finding the right mix of health care providers, cost and effectiveness, and the quality and safety of care.

The nurse supply

Nurses worldwide are an intrinsic part of caring for people in hospitals and are the backbone of community health and chronic long-term care. However, a shortage of professional nurses in most countries is threatening the adequacy, quality, and safety of care. The shortage is partly brought about by increasing demand from the aging population worldwide and changes in acute care delivery models in some countries, such as the use of mostly registered nurses rather than licensed practical nurses and aides in US hospitals.

Although the USA has a larger supply than many other countries, its nurse shortage is expected to become a crisis over the next 50 years. Increases in patient acuity in hospitals, as advanced technology sustains the lives of patients who a few years ago would have died, means more patients require highly intense care. Hospitals have responded to the growing number of acutely ill patients and soaring costs by reducing lengths of stays. This, in turn, means that a larger proportion of inpatients depend totally on advanced nursing care, which fuels the demand for a higher nurse–patient ratio.

In other countries, hospitals often keep patients longer, enabling them to heal and regain their ability to care for themselves. Nursing care may be less intensive, but generally there also are fewer available nurses; staff nurses are equally if not more stressed and overworked than their US counterparts. These factors, along with stagnant compensation in many cases, lead to burn-out, dissatisfaction, and high turnover.

The nurse shortage is closely linked to four other issues: nursing education, unlicensed nursing care providers, nurse migration, and maldistribution.

Nursing education

Educating nurses is expensive and requires adequate numbers of highly trained and experienced faculty. Nursing faculty are also in short supply. In the USA, the average age of nursing school faculty members is 52, the proportion reaching retirement age is growing rapidly, and fewer younger nurses with a graduate education are joining the faculty ranks (American Association of Colleges of Nursing 2005). Using practicing nurses as clinical teachers compensates in part for the faculty shortage, but increasing workloads constrain their capacity for teaching and supervising students.

One probable cause of the faculty shortage is that nurses with the advanced degrees necessary to teach have discovered they can earn more money in the service sector than in education. In many countries, skilled nurses are unlikely to leave their high-paying positions to pursue higher education, while nurses who invest the time it takes to obtain an advanced degree have less practical experience. The situation calls for government assistance and policies to balance salaries across settings. It also calls for research that would shed light on the financial and social aspects of nurses' job choices, and guide changes in nursing education policy.

Unlicensed care providers

Since professional nursing education began a century and a half ago, discussion has focused on the use of lesser-trained and unlicensed care providers. Various types and levels of nursing care providers – some with less education and knowledge than others – help stretch the workforce to meet demand. This discussion must continue and include the overarching concern for the quality and safety of care.

Research conducted mostly in North America, the UK, and Western Europe has demonstrated the importance of sufficient numbers of registered nurses (RNs) in hospitals. But there has been little research in other countries, or in other practice settings globally, linking RN staffing and the quality of care. Nor has much research addressed the mix of professional and non-professional nursing care providers in hospitals and community settings that would be of greatest benefit to health care consumers. Trained lay providers guided by professional nurses could make a big difference in extending the benefits of basic health care. Creating, implementing, and evaluating care delivery models that incorporate a mix of providers to promote healthy child development, maternal health, disease prevention education, and more would shed light on the value of this approach. Studies also need to determine the supervision, support, and protocols for non-professionals that would be necessary to provide effective and safe care (Holzemer 2008).

Migration

Developed countries recruit RNs from developing countries with the promise of higher salaries and better living conditions (Kingma 2006). Developing countries within the same geographic region also recruit experienced nurses from each other. This benefits individual nurses and the nations to which they emigrate, but it causes severe shortages in the home countries. Research on this subject for the purpose of policy development is crucial. The extent to which health care investments affect a nation's production and retention of trained health care workers warrants examination. In addition, there is a need to develop strategies that benefit both the sending and receiving countries and that promote a sharing of knowledge and experience gained from such intermingling. Finally, assessments of working conditions – and the development of policies related to those conditions – would elucidate the forces spurring migration and help stabilize the nurse workforce worldwide (International Council of Nursing [ICN] 2007a).

It is possible to shape migration as a win–win proposition for the sending and receiving countries. Nurses who work abroad take their education and experience with them, which, depending on the strengths and limitations of one's education and experience, can be positive or negative for these nations. Research to identify such strengths and limitations could be useful, and compensating the sending countries for the resources they invest in nursing education would help balance this inequity. All countries and nurses involved in migration would benefit from systems that support nurses who leave for discreet and limited periods of time, then return home to share their knowledge and experience with colleagues.

Maldistribution

Inadequate distribution of nurses within a country poses a major problem for its health care system and nursing education. Nurses are more likely to work in urban than in remote rural areas, attracted by higher salaries, more opportunities for continuing education, and modern facilities. The fewer health care resources, less desirable working conditions, and demands for public-health and primary-care competencies in rural areas exacerbate this problem. An increasing number of private, for-profit agencies – usually located in cities – recruit experienced nurses from public and rural institutions that have fewer resources.

Research would guide successful policies for recruiting and retaining nurses in rural areas and public institutions where they are needed most.

Working conditions for nurses also warrant attention. Such conditions, as well as workplace design, the way work is delegated, the actual workload, and staffing balance, all affect nurses' productivity. A question for researchers is: What steps would promote the best care for all patients? Higher nursing salaries? A better work environment? Better socioeconomic conditions generally? Greater nurse control over clinical practice and working conditions? Other factors?

To combat the ever-increasing nurse shortage worldwide, it is necessary to intervene in workforce policy and planning, enhance education capacity, create positive practice environments, improve organizational performance, and address migration, maldistribution, and issues related to nurse recruitment and retention (ICN 2006).

Measuring performance, productivity, and value

A necessary foundation for research on nursing education, nurse supply, skill mix, working conditions, and other factors is a clear consensus across disciplines about the nature of nursing care and medical care, and the best ways to measure performance and productivity. Two long-sought goals are to clarify nurse roles and develop valid measures of their workload. Western countries have made progress in measuring hospital workload, but there has been little progress in other areas of the globe and in other care settings.

Although nurses are the central caregivers in most settings, researchers need to examine the role of each member of the health care team to clarify nurses' contributions. Before investigators study the best way to structure teams that provide acute, long-term, and community-based care, and community health education, they must learn which physician and nurse responsibilities and tasks could be delegated to others. Research on how well other providers handle these responsibilities and tasks would follow. Such studies would promote workforce planning, adequate training, and appropriate policy to maximize the potential of health care.

Agreement on and use of a common nursing database would be a crucial step toward successful international research on nursing productivity and effectiveness. There are several different database standards, but none dominates. European and Asian researchers tend to use the International Classification for Nursing Practice (ICN 2007b), while those in the USA and a few other countries prefer databases known as NANDA (from the North American Nursing Diagnosis Association), NIC (Nursing Interventions Classification), and NOC (Nursing Outcomes Classification) (Allred et al. 2004; Van Krogh et al. 2005). Difficulties reaching consensus on data definitions and standards have greatly impeded national and cross-national research. There has been progress in terms of identifying and agreeing on the data necessary for acute care studies, but much remains to be done (Van den Heede et al. 2007).

Determining the right provider mix

Determining the appropriate mix of providers must occur on at least two levels. The first and higher level entails macro workforce planning and deployment, in which governing entities decide how best to invest in the preparation of nurses, physicians, and other health care providers. This level involves policy decisions about two issues: balancing the scope of practice for each discipline with citizens' need for services that fit into the different roles and contributions of each discipline, and investing resources productively. Comparative international research on the health of populations in areas with different provider mixes would guide decisions about appropriate resource investments.

Beyond decisions about the relative number of people that should be educated in various health care disciplines, countries should determine how they will encourage deployment of providers to areas with the greatest need. Macro health outcomes studies examining the impact that different provider mixes have on the health of populations would be very useful, as would research on differential compensation for professionals who accept and remain in jobs in under-served areas.

At the second, more micro level, a subject that warrants study is the appropriate mix of nursing care providers within an institution or community. In an era of increasing shortages of RNs, it is important to know how to provide nursing care in an efficient, safe, and effective manner, and how to create and organize health care delivery in ways that maximize the benefits of RNs and unlicensed nurses while maintaining quality.

Another topic for research is identifying the right mix of providers to meet general health care needs. Yet to be developed and tested are the types of education and skill necessary to accomplish this, and ways to extend the use of professionally trained nurses to the care that physicians have traditionally provided. This will require setting aside territorial squabbles among disciplines in order to bring the best care possible to the largest number of people at the lowest cost. Nurses, physicians, and others must rethink how they communicate with and respect each other when, as teams, they plan and deliver care.

Cost-effectiveness

Health care policy-makers seek knowledge about the cost of treatments and procedures, and the effectiveness of services, including basic care for illnesses and accidents. However, most cost-effectiveness studies are more narrowly focused on new technologies, surgical or medical advances, or disease detection. Furthermore, studies that examine effectiveness at a basic level do not specify trade-offs between investment in primary preventive care and secondary or tertiary acute care. And cost-effectiveness research rarely includes general nursing care. In reviewing the few nursing-related cost studies that have been published in the USA, Rothberg et al. (2005) concluded that spending more on hospital nursing care would be a good investment. A broader approach to national and international cost-effectiveness research would help guide nurses as they care for the sick, promote health, and try to prevent disease.

Research to address these issues must be at the macro level, include studies of single countries and studies that compare countries, and be conducted by nurses and others with training in health services and health economics. A crucial emphasis is the cost-effectiveness implications of:

(1) The mix of nursing care providers (licensed, unlicensed, professional, lay) and health care providers (physicians, nurses, others);
(2) The supply, deployment, and retention of all health care providers; and
(3) The allocation of providers across acute care, long-term care, and community settings.

International studies can best demonstrate the strengths and weaknesses of various models for funding health care. Excellent examples of such research are Retzlaff-Roberts et al. (2003) and Schoen et al. (2005). However, these studies did not differentiate nursing care from other types of care. International research on financing models that account for nursing care would be very useful as countries worldwide struggle to provide essential services.

Care quality and safety

In all health care settings globally, the challenge is to balance the quality of care and patient safety with costs. Table 5.1 summarizes the priorities that the USA, UK, and Canada place on quality and safety.

Patient safety depends on high-quality care from nurses and others, and on excellent communication and teamwork among providers. Errors, a major cause of safety risks, involve improper actions – for example, those related to

Table 5.1 Health care quality and safety priorities.

USA	UK	Canada
Care that is: • *Safe* (avoids injuries) • *Effective*, based on scientifically proven benefits. Effective care also means not providing services to people who are unlikely to benefit from them • *Patient-centered*. Such care respects and responds to the preferences, needs, and values of individual patients • *Timely*. Care should reduce waiting and harmful delays • *Efficient*. It avoids wasting equipment, supplies, ideas, and energy • *Equitable*. The quality of care should not vary due to gender, ethnicity, geography, and socioeconomic status	Emphasis is on: • Reducing variation in adherence to best practices • Increasing clinical accountability • Spawning national clinical databases • Developing clear policies, effective processes, and appropriate incentives • Fostering a team approach to care • Spurring robust assessment and widespread roll-out of approved technologies • Enabling health care providers to report and systematically learn from adverse events	Recognizing the inevitability of human error, emphasis is on: • Evidence-based practice • A team approach to care • Comprehensive identification of hazards • Not blaming individuals for errors • Shifting away from health care's traditional hierarchical structure • Cost-effective and evidence-based safety initiatives and standards • Public disclosure and transparency of hospital adverse events • Patient-centered care • Non-punitive reporting • Healthy work environments

Sources: USA, Institute of Medicine (2001); UK, Department of Health (2006); and Canada, National Steering Committee on Patient Safety (2002).

prescribing and administering medications, performing procedures, and diagnosing problems – as well as omissions, such as not providing care that is known to be effective and not controlling hazards. Some threats, such as falls, skin breakdown, and nosocomial infections, are more responsive to nursing care than others, such as surgical mishaps. Medication safety is a paramount concern; the Institute of Medicine (2007) estimated that preventable medication errors harm as many as 1.5 million Americans each year.

Two of the biggest health care problems worldwide are the spread of communicable disease and infections related to treatment. The international patient safety movement has focused first on preventing nosocomial infections by aggressively promoting handwashing (World Health Organization 2006b). Research has demonstrated that higher RN staffing is associated with lower nosocomial infection rates (Hugonnet et al. 2004).

Ideally, recommendations by groups in the USA and elsewhere for improving the quality and safety of care are based on evidence. But such evidence is sparse. This suggests that vast resources are being spent on improving quality and safety without data to support the likelihood that certain types of initiatives will succeed. More research is necessary.

There are international efforts to improve quality of care through evidence-based practice. The Cochrane collection[1] in the UK, for example, gathers and integrates research knowledge regarding specific care activities. The Joanna Briggs Institute[2] promotes evidence-based nursing practice at hospitals in Australia and a number of other countries.

Four reviews (Lang et al. 2004; Blegen 2006; Kane et al. 2007; Hughes 2008) summarize current knowledge on the relationship between nurse staffing levels and the quality and safety of patient care in hospitals, and point to particular needs for future research.

Conclusions

Major nursing-related issues need further research, efforts that would proceed more easily if there were standard data definitions and databases. International scholars have addressed research priorities for nursing in the last decade. Topping the list are the safety and quality of patient care (Yin et al. 2000; Moreno-Casbas et al. 2001; French et al. 2002; Kim et al. 2002; Drennan et al. 2007). Second on the list are care delivery concerns: nurse staffing, working conditions, and organization of care (Yin et al. 2000; Ross et al. 2004; Annells et al. 2005; Drennan et al. 2007). Yin et al. (2000) and Kim et al. (2002) cited the cost-effectiveness of nursing care as an important issue, and Van den Heede et al. (2007) mentioned standardized measures of nurse staffing and patient outcomes related to nursing care.

National and international efforts to equalize nursing care supply and demand require research on nurse migration and distribution within and between countries. Working conditions would also be a fruitful focus of studies which could inform institutional and national policy. Finally, to promote delivery of appropriate and affordable care to all citizens of all nations, research and consensus-building regarding the roles of health care providers and the best way to structure teams to deliver services effectively and efficiently are central to progress.

Notes

1   www.cochrane.org
2   www.joannabriggs.edu.au

References

Allred, S.K., Smith, K.F. & Flowers, L. (2004) Electronic implementation of national nursing standards: NANDA, NOC, and NIC as an effective teaching tool. *Journal of Healthcare Information Management* **18**(4), 56–60.

American Association of Colleges of Nursing (2005) *Faculty shortages in baccalaureate and graduate nursing programs: Scope of the problem and strategies for expanding the supply.* Washington, D.C.: American Association of Colleges of Nursing.

Annells, M., DeRoche, M., Koch, T., Lewin, G. & Lucke, J. (2005) A Delphi study of district nursing research priorities in Australia. *Applied Nursing Research* **18**(1), 36–43.

Blegen, M.A. (2006) Patient safety in hospital acute care units. *Annual Review of Nursing Research* **24**, 103–125.

Department of Health (2006) *Good doctors, safer patients: Proposals to strengthen the system to assure and improve the performance of doctors and to protect the safety of patients.* Norwich: Department of Health.

Drennan, J., Mehan, T., Kemple, M., Johnson, M., Treacy, M. & Butler, M. (2007) Nursing research priorities for Ireland. *Journal of Nursing Scholarship* **39**(4), 298–305.

French, P., Ho, Y. & Lee, L. (2002) A Delphi survey of evidence-based nursing priorities in Hong Kong. *Journal of Nursing Management* **10**(5), 265–273.

Holzemer, W.L. (2008) Building a global nursing workforce. *International Nursing Review* **5**(3), 1241–1242.

Hughes, R. (2008) *Patient safety and quality: An evidence-based handbook for nurses.* AHRQ Publication No. 07-00151. Rockville, MD: Agency for Healthcare Research and Quality.

Hugonnet, S., Harbarth, S., Sax, H., Duncan, R. & Pittet, D. (2004) Nursing resources: A major determinant of nosocomial infection? *Current Opinion in Infectious Diseases,* **17**, 329–333.

Institute of Medicine (2001) *Crossing the quality chasm: A new health system for the 21st century.* Washington D.C.: National Academies Press.

Institute of Medicine (2007) *Preventing medication errors.* Washington D.C.: National Academies Press.

International Council of Nurses (2006) *The global nursing shortage: Priority areas for intervention.* Geneva: International Council of Nurses.

International Council of Nurses (2007a) *Positive practice environments: Quality workplaces = quality patient care.* Geneva: International Council of Nurses.

International Council of Nurses (2007b) *International classification for nursing practice.* Geneva: International Council of Nurses.

Kane, R.L., Shamliyan, T., Mueller, C., Duval, S. & Wilt, T. (2007) The association of registered nurse staffing levels and patient outcomes: Systematic review and meta-analysis. *Medical Care* **45**(12), 1195–1204.

Kim, M.J., Oh, E., Kim, C., Yoo, J. & Ko, I. (2002) Priorities for nursing research in Korea. *Journal of Nursing Scholarship* **34**(4), 307–312.

Kingma, M. (2006) *Nurses on the Move: Migration and the global economy.* Ithaca, New York: Cornell University Press.

Lang, T., Hodge, M., Olson, V., Romano, P. & Kravitz, R. (2004) Nurse–patient ratios: A systematic review of the effects of nurse staffing on patients, nurse employee, and hospital outcomes. *Journal of Nursing Administration* **34**(7/8), 326–337.

Moreno-Casbas, T., Martin-Arribas, C., Orts-Cortes, I. & Comet-Cortes, P. (2001) Identification of priorities for nursing research in Spain: A Delphi study. *Journal of Advanced Nursing* **35**(6), 857–863.

National Steering Committee on Patient Safety (2002) *Building a safer system: A national integrated strategy for improving patient safety in Canadian health care.* Ottawa: National Steering Committee on Patient Safety.

Retzlaff-Roberts, D., Chang, C.F. & Rubin, R.M. (2003) Technical efficiency in the use of health care resources: A comparison of OECD countries. *Health Policy* **69**(1), 55–72.

Ross, F., Smith, E., Mackenzie, A. & Masterson, A. (2004) Identifying research priorities in nursing and midwifery service delivery and organization. *International Journal of Nursing Studies* **41**(5), 547–558.

Rothberg, M., Abraham, I., Lindenauer, P. & Rose, D. (2005) Improving nurse-to-patient staffing ratios as a cost-effective safety intervention. *Medical Care* **43**(8), 785–791.

Schoen, C., Osborn, R., Huynh, P.T., Doty, M., Zapert, K., Peugh, J., et al. (2005) Taking the pulse of health care systems: Experiences of patients with health problems in six countries. *Health Affairs* **W5**, 509–525.

Van den Heede, K., Clarke, S., Sermeus, W., Vleugels, A. & Aikin, L. (2007) International experts' perspectives on the state of the nurse staffing and patient outcomes literature: Results of a Delphi study. *Journal of Nursing Scholarship* **39**(4), 290–297.

Van Krogh, G., Dale, C. & Naden, D. (2005) A framework for integrating NANDA, NIC, and NOC terminology in electronic patient records. *Journal of Nursing Scholarship* **37**(3), 275–281.

World Health Organization (2006a) *The world health report 2006: Working together for health.* Geneva: WHO.

World Health Organization (2006b) *World alliance for patient safety: Forward programme 2006–2007.* Geneva: WHO.

Yin, T., Hsu, N., Tsai, S., Wang, B., Shaw, F., Shih, F., et al. (2000) Priority setting for nursing research in the Republic of China. *Journal of Advanced Nursing* **32**(1), 19–27.

Chapter 6
Building professional nursing

June Webber

Introduction

The nursing profession has become well-established in a number of countries around the world over the last century. In the course of its evolution, the profession has had to navigate increasingly complex issues related to global change.

Today's 'modern world system,' a term coined by Immanuel Wallerstein in 1974, features intertwining flows of communications, populations, cultures, financial markets, and politics. The 'overarching processes and transformations [operating] at a global level' have an impact on everyone's reality, introducing or influencing conditions and variables at the local, national, and regional levels (Cohen & Kennedy 2000, p. 10). These conditions and variables affect nursing, health systems, and health outcomes. Health systems worldwide face many challenges to their effectiveness, including an increasing shortage of health providers, a growing tide of environmental health issues, and persistent and widening health inequities fueled by poverty. The health challenges are wide-ranging – from infectious and transmittable diseases such as HIV/AIDS, malaria, tuberculosis, dengue fever, and chronic illnesses, to the needs of aging populations, mothers and children, the socially marginalized, and victims of natural disasters.

The modern global system means nurses must deal with a complexity of health systems, health and professional issues, and gender issues central to their autonomy and self-image. While these conditions threaten nurses' ability to practice, they also present enormous opportunities to apply research, knowledge, and innovations. Concerned about its growth, contribution, relevance, and sustainability, the profession needs to be aware of global trends as well as local sociopolitical forces so it can effectively adapt and take a leadership role in addressing global and local health imperatives through evidence-based innovations. In addition, it must build cross-border partnerships aimed at communicating influential trends, building the discipline, and supporting organizational and professional capacity.

Nursing has a formidable role in health systems globally. Networking enables the profession to grow and widely disseminate its scientific foundations and practice base. However, this growth has been uneven, given the diverse and often inequitable realities in many regions. As nurse researchers contribute evidence demonstrating that educational preparation and workplace resources are linked with health outcomes, a growing ethos and practice of global social responsibility is being integrated into international efforts to strengthen nursing in low and middle-income countries, creating a new nursing globalism.

Understanding this concept, which is based on the values and beliefs inherent to social justice, requires a broader analysis of where the nursing profession fits into global trends and issues. What are the past and present realities that influence nursing's contribution to health care? What are the key building blocks of a strong nursing profession – one that advances knowledge, innovates, establishes policy, and delivers services with the goal of strengthening health systems and improving patient outcomes? What role should the profession have in redressing inequities encountered by nurses worldwide?

This chapter considers nursing's development in the context of rapid globalization, highlighting the historical, political, and economic factors that have made this development uneven. It also identifies the building blocks of nursing professionalism and the central role of related organizations in advancing the profession nationally and internationally. Finally, the chapter explores mechanisms to support professional development in low and middle-income countries and introduces the concept of a new nursing globalism, which reflects an international collegiality based on cooperative and equity-minded health partnerships.

From early industrialization to market domination

The world has experienced a relatively rapid evolution in the way political and financial entities are organized and relate to each other. Inspired by the French Revolution and accelerated by industrialization, nation states have replaced local domains, principalities, and kingdoms that once governed society and the production and distribution of wealth. The domination of capitalism as an economic organizing principle has escalated through the emergence of transnational corporations, which have become somewhat overbearing players in global affairs. This capitalistic system, according to Canadian activist Naomi Klein (2007), generates tremendous profits for corporations but leaves many people in misery.

Over the last century, the world has experienced a dramatic shift in mechanisms central to governance and economic forces – in the way the production of goods and services is organized and negotiated – within a framework of accelerated connectivity, or 'globalization.' As an operating principle, globalization refers to the process of integration. Generically, the term encompasses 'all those processes by which the peoples of the world are incorporated into a single society, global society' (Cohen & Kennedy 2000, p. 24). It entails an accelerated exchange of information, knowledge, cultural innovations, and influences.

A driving force behind this trend is economic globalization, in which the world's economies become increasingly integrated as capital, services, technology, and labor move among them, leading to globally based economic decisions (Labonté & Schrecker 2007). A related trend is deregulation of national economies to accelerate the movement of goods and services, enabling banks and corporations to maximize profits. A third trend is the widening gap between rich and poor within and between nations. The gap creates greater inequities along the lines of gender, race/ethnicity, and class; as a result, disparities have grown dramatically in the last few decades (Cohen & Kennedy 2000; Labonté & Schrecker 2007), thus exacerbating uneven development worldwide.

Nations gain recognition from other nations when they are accepted into international decision-making entities – the United Nations, the Group of 8, the International Monetary Fund, the World Bank, the World Trade Organization – that consider, align, process, and set policy directions and account for global economic, political, and social interests. The number of nation states seeking global recognition so they can inform international policy-making continues to grow as more sub-national religious and ethnic identities seek autonomy and recognition.

The accelerated movement of economies and major technologic advances, along with intensifying global competition, has caused enormous changes in the workplace. As markets adapt by adopting more flexible and informal labor practices, the result has been greater economic insecurity and challenges for vulnerable groups, particularly women, as they encounter the internationalization, feminization, and casualization of work (Cohen & Kennedy 2000). When employees have a choice in the matter, casualization – re-employing regular workers on a casual or short-term basis – may offer flexibility. However, the trend has been toward imposed casualization characterized by intermittent work, inconsistent work hours, and little access to the rights and benefits of permanent employment.

While the surge of post-World War II capitalism increased the focus on markets as an indicator of national advancement, health gained recognition as a global good and – through the Universal Declaration of Human Rights, reinforced in the 1978 Declaration of Alma-Ata – a global right. A 2001 report to the World Health Organization (WHO) by the Commission on Macroeconomics and Health illustrated the inextricable link between health and development. The report's principal author, economist Jeffrey Sachs, explained how good health and economic development benefit each other. He asserted that millions of lives could be saved, poverty could be reduced, economic development would ensue, and global security could be more easily promoted by 'extending the coverage of crucial health services, including a relatively small number of specific interventions, to the world's poor' (Sachs 2001, p. 1).

Over the years, the WHO has persistently declared its global commitment to health equity. In 2005, it formed the Commission on Social Determinants of Health on the premise that understanding the social determinants of health – the conditions in which people live and work, which affect their opportunities to lead healthy lives – is perhaps the most effective way to reduce inequities while progressing toward health for all (Labonté & Schrecker 2007).

Researchers and public health advocates maintain that the underlying social determinants of health are the best predictors of an individual's and a population's health (Raphael 2003; Marmot & Wilkinson 2006). Socioeconomic status is by far the most significant predictor of health, and thus poses greater health challenges and worse health for the world's poor (WHO 2007).

Indeed, men and women worldwide have consistently ranked good health as their highest priority (Sachs 2001). Health is at the foundation of one's capacity to learn, live, work, love, and care. Sachs found that societies bearing a heavy disease burden have succumbed to a range of challenges to economic progress. This consequence is most severe in impoverished countries struggling with communicable diseases, high maternal and infant mortality rates, and malnutrition, which inevitably affect the poor more profoundly.

Market demand for new efficiencies may pressure health systems to treat and process illnesses mechanistically rather than humanistically. Such an approach to patient care often undermines the knowledge and evidence that support professional practice and health system needs. According to Sullivan and Benner (2005, p. 78), 'professionals are major contributors to the prosperity and high level of technical development in all advanced societies, yet today's pressured drive toward accelerated information and communications technology driven by "frictionless capitalism" threatens to erode the capacity of nursing professionals to apply their knowledge and expertise within a framework of judgment and social integrity.' The question, then, is how does the nursing profession situate itself amid global trends that are counter-intuitive to its core ethos?

Building the nursing profession

Nursing has made dramatic strides toward professional recognition, although the journey has not been easy and political, social, and economic challenges remain. The profession has established a growing body of knowledge that is inherent in educational and credentialing standards in many parts of the world. Nurses also have more diverse and advanced roles in many practice environments than they did in the past. Recognition of these roles means more autonomy and stature for the profession.

The tenets of nursing as an occupation for women date to the theoretical and practical contributions of Florence Nightingale in the late 19th century. The chief criterion then was that 'to be a good nurse, one must be a good woman' (Marks 1994, p. 4). Victorian England was at the height of its imperial dominance amid a rapidly growing industrialism in which an industrial workforce was central to production and profit. Although class, gender, and, increasingly, ethnicity determined one's place in society, industrialism's rise set the stage for formalization of professional groups.

Visionary nurse leaders were intent on gaining recognition and legitimacy for their profession by distinguishing it from the powerful medical profession. One of the most influential leaders, Ethel Bedford-Fenwick, was instrumental in establishing the British Nursing Association. Her lobbying for the professionalization of nursing shifted some control of the profession by hospital authorities to nurse associations, which became responsible for setting educational standards and compulsory registration (Witz 1992; Marks 1994; Bowden 1997).

Educator Abraham Flexner helped align nursing with the tenets of professionalism by, among other things, identifying three core elements of professionalism: a specialized body of knowledge specific to the occupational practice, self-regulatory power, and state recognition (McCoppin & Gardner 1994). His work was grounded in efforts by the medical profession to establish criteria that would give it autonomy and elite status for physicians (Marks 1994). The attributes of professionalism that Flexner described have endured as goals for nursing.

However, a number of enduring occupational ambiguities undermine perceptions of the nursing profession. Indeed, many researchers have argued that the gendered nature of nursing has persistently usurped recognition of nurses and their professional autonomy. The issue of gender as it relates to professional recognition is illustrated in discourses about 'care' and 'virtue' (Gilligan 1982; Rispel & Schneider 1989; Armstrong 1993; Marks 1994; Bowden 1997; Nelson & Gordon 2006). Such attitudes may have displaced recognition of nurses' knowledge and expertise, and provided a familiar terrain for undervaluing their role (Gordon 2005; Clark 2006; Nelson 2006; Nelson & Gordon 2006); resulted in persistent subordination of nurses to physicians in the biomedical model (Witz 1992); or led to inadequate resources and clinical support, eroding nurses' capacity to apply knowledge and clinical skills effectively (Armstrong 1993). For nurses, the consequences are poor remuneration in many countries, lack of autonomy and voice, and poor stature and social value.

Health systems worldwide are struggling with shortages of human and material resources that impede access to care and effective response to health priorities. Although nurses are well-educated and constitute the majority of providers, they are not generally consulted about solutions to health system problems, even though, paradoxically, they are the most trusted of providers. In many countries, unregulated caregivers are being trained – a quick fix for the health provider shortage that, absent adequate integration and mentorship of these workers, may threaten health outcomes.

Nursing knowledge and practice were regionalized in the 19th and 20th centuries as a result of imperial and colonial forms of development. As the nursing profession took shape in countries with diverse economies, social structures, and politics, its organization, characteristics, and place within health systems became contextually distinctive. For example, South Africa was among the first countries to form a national nurse association and affiliate with the International Council of Nurses when the council was established in the late 19th century. At that time, nursing adhered to the precepts of Victorian England; entry into the profession in South Africa was restricted to women of English heritage. Afrikaaner, Indian, and African women did not gain entry until later. As industrialization escalated in the 1940s, a growing working class of black people needed health care providers. Consequently, nursing in South Africa absorbed more black women who previously had been barred. While educational content was consistent across the board, racial disparities arose in terms of how South African nurses were educated and remunerated, the types of work they performed, and where they were permitted to work (Marks 1994; Rispel 1995; Webber 2001).

Yet, despite the apartheid policies of the late 1940s, the nursing profession stayed abreast of global developments. Its most formidable architect, Charlotte Searle, became the first nurse in South Africa to earn a PhD. Although she prepared and inspired a formidable network of nurse scientists who contributed knowledge and expertise, most black nurses lacked access to professional education and exposure to scientific practice until the country liberalized its apartheid laws in the mid-1980s. Today, South Africa still is redressing the damage that apartheid caused to its health care system as the nursing profession seeks to strengthen its leadership and research capacity, and to retain members.

Although there has been considerable global progress in building the profession, advances still depend on national context. Historical, political, and economic realities have led to disproportionate investments in health systems, and to insufficient educational preparation, advancement, and recognition of practitioners. In many countries, one consequence of economic disparities and factors that create structural or social instability at the national or regional level is uneven development of health systems and the nursing profession.

Autonomy through knowledge, self-regulation, and affiliation

In many parts of the world, nurses have achieved a status as the health care providers with the most diversified skills and are authorized to practice autonomously, regardless of the complexity of care they provide or how predictable the outcomes may be (Canadian Nurses Association [CNA] 2002a). As a result of globalization of nursing knowledge, nurses worldwide now have the necessary skills, knowledge, and judgment to assess patients comprehensively, use scientific knowledge to interpret and sythesize information, anticipate positive and negative outcomes, and provide therapy to patients (CNA 2002a). Nursing has gained recognition in national and regional settings, thanks to self-regulation, registration, licensure, and affiliation with professional organizations. Such affiliation makes nurses part of a larger community and invests them in the direction the profession must take and in the health priorities it must address.

Knowledge and attributes

A growing body of evidence has guided the formation of nursing attributes and parameters for performance in the context of evolving health systems and priorities. The contributions of nurse researchers and professional organizations to the development of entry level competencies are well-documented.

Like other professionals, nurses aspire to apply and gauge their knowledge, values, and behaviors. The Registered Nurses' Association of Ontario (RNAO) (2007) has identified attributes it deems central to the profession. Based on an extensive literature review and broad consultation with nurse leaders and practitioners, the association delineated a number of important attributes and indicators that should serve as best practice guidelines for, and measures of, professional practice (Table 6.1). By framing these attributes in the context of work environments, the association has reinforced the influence of health system or practice setting factors, such as funding or other resources (RNAO 2007).

Today, building the profession includes finding ways to disseminate knowledge globally and integrate relevant evidence into nursing practice. The International Council of Nurses has a key role in this regard by enlisting diverse constituencies to develop policy positions, standards, and codes of practice. Its leadership as a normative body enables the profession to speak with one voice.

Self-regulation

Professional practice includes the application of scientific and evidence-based knowledge and technical skills, and a commitment to practice ethically according to

Table 6.1 Attributes and indicators of professionalism in nursing.

Attribute	Indicators
Knowledge	• Theoretical, practical, and clinical knowledge • Able to apply that knowledge • Uses a theoretical and/or evidence-based rationale for practice • Synthesizes and uses information from a variety of sources • Shares knowledge with, or communicates it to colleagues, clients, family members, and others to continually improve care and health outcomes
Spirit of enquiry	• Open-minded and eager to explore new knowledge • Asks questions that lead to new, or the refinement of existing, knowledge • Defines patterns of responses from clients and stakeholders, and their context • Committed to lifelong learning
Accountability	• Understands the meaning of self-regulation and its implications for practice • Uses legislation, standards of practice, and a code of ethics to clarify one's scope of practice • Committed to working with clients and families to achieve desired outcomes • Actively engages in advancing the quality of care • Recognizes personal capabilities, knowledge, and types of expertise that need to be developed
Autonomy	• Works independently and makes decisions within one's appropriate scope of practice • Recognizes relational autonomy and the effects that context and relationships have on it • Is aware of barriers and constraints that may interfere with one's autonomy, and seeks ways to remedy them
Advocacy	• Understands the client's perspective • Helps the client meet learning needs • Is involved in professional practice initiatives and activities to enhance health care • Knowledgeable about policies that affect the delivery of health care
Innovation and visionary thinking	• Fosters a culture of innovation to enhance client/family outcomes • Shows initiative for new ideas and gets involved by taking action • Influences the future of nursing, delivery of health care, and the health care system
Collegiality and collaboration	• Develops collaborative partnerships in a professional context • Is a mentor to nurses, nursing students, and colleagues to enhance and support professional growth • Acknowledges and recognizes the interdependence of care providers
Ethics and values	• Knowledgeable about ethical values, concepts, and decision-making • Is able to identify ethical concerns, issues, and dilemmas • Applies knowledge of nursing ethics to making, and acting upon, decisions • Is able to collect and use information from various sources for ethical decision-making • Collaborates with colleagues to develop and maintain a practice environment that supports nurses and respects their ethical and professional responsibilities • Thinks critically about ethical issues in clinical and professional practice

a social contract between nursing and society. A function of this contract is self-regulation, a right that society gives to the profession to decide who has the necessary knowledge, judgment, attributes, and skills to provide safe, competent, and ethical care (CNA 2007a).

The core elements of self-regulation are:

- *Licensure and registration.* In many instances, the title 'registered nurse' is protected. Only nurses who are licensed by a regulatory body can practice;
- *Ethical values.* The profession's codified values and standards of ethical performance delineate the basic knowledge nurses must have and their ethical responsibilities to the public;
- *Standards of practice and entry-level competencies.* The profession sets baseline standards of knowledge, judgment, attributes, and skills to ensure that registrants have entry-level competencies to practice safely and ethically in a designated role and setting. These standards are the platform that support a practitioner's progression from novice to expert;
- *Educational preparation.* The theoretical and practical content, experience, and mentorship in an approved nursing education program prepare students for safe, ethical, and competent practice after graduation. Increasingly, countries worldwide want nurses who enter the profession to have a baccalaureate degree; and
- *Continuing competence and development of expertise.* Professional affiliation connotes a commitment to lifelong learning. Nurses increase their knowledge and skills through experience, formal learning, and evidence-based practice. Exposure to evolving technologies, specialty certification, ongoing academic education, mentorship, and the use of best-practice guidelines aid this process.

Regulatory bodies are responsible for controlling entry into the profession, the content and parameters of nursing education, and professional conduct. Professions and their practitioners, unlike businesses, pledge to protect people in vulnerable situations. They are 'communities of living craft-knowledge that have become self-reflective about their practices' whose knowledge in the regulation domain is 'the collective possession [of the profession and] also a social asset of which the organised profession is the collective steward' (Sullivan & Benner 2005, p. 80).

According to Sullivan and Benner (2005), the social reciprocity central to a profession's mandate to vigilantly safeguard populations and the individuals it serves is civic professionalism. They note that work environments and practice settings increasingly dominated by the private market take a more narrowly focused, business-like approach. Although professions in the private and public domains sell their services, nurses' expert services and values constitute an essential public good. Importantly, the notion of civic professionalism qualifies the way professionals interpret their role relative to society and the community, and is consistent with the fabric of social responsibility discussed earlier.

Professional associations

Professionals are key to the development of the theoretical foundations, technical know-how, and technological innovations necessary to support local-to-global economies. However, impatient with the pace of economic development amid globalization, many developing countries with weak health care systems seek a quick fix by importing unregulated health workers who are not part of a comprehensive, interdisciplinary, and professional framework.

Given the increasing global interconnectedness and complexities that impact health, health systems, and providers, many nursing leaders say the profession must rethink its core elements (Villeneuve & MacDonald 2006), strengthen nurses' capacity and ability to 'function within an increasingly dysfunctional system' (Nelson 2006, p. 87), and better position nurses to influence policy (Rains & Barton-Kriese 2001; Hughes 2005; Nicklin & Stipich 2005; Welchman & Griener 2005; CNA 2006a; Oulton 2006; Shaw 2007).

Now more than ever, professional nurse associations have a vital role in bringing nurses together locally, nationally, and internationally to identify priorities and obstacles that prevent better health outcomes, analyze trends and clarify policy gaps, generate research questions aimed at data collection, and use evidence to develop options and innovate. They also have a role in developing collective power and asserting the profession's knowledge and expertise in strengthening health systems. One of their tasks is building the legitimacy of nursing in addressing the many complex challenges to better health outcomes and equipping the profession with the resources, evidence, and networks it needs to meet those challenges.

An investigation by Wynd (2003) of factors that affect professionalism in nursing explored the attitudes of professionals and their links with associations. She determined that active engagement in an association's decisions – attending meetings, joining committees, and staying abreast of the professional literature – was an essential way for professionals to become socialized. Her study concluded that affiliation with a professional association is a predictor of professionalism.

Nurse associations are social structures guided by a vision and mission. They set corresponding goals for the results they want to achieve. Associations may have complex governance structures that identify policy and program priorities calling for leadership skills based on strong knowledge and a capacity to influence, persuade, and form and collaborate within strategic alliances. Unlike businesses, which seek profits, professional associations measure achievement in terms of progress toward their objectives.

The focus and orientation of professional associations vary, depending on their purpose and the members they serve. Those that cater to members may concentrate on the interests and imperatives of a particular domain, such as advancing nursing practice, education, research, administration, or health policy. A broader professional scope may involve providing continuing education, certification, or other member services. Or it may extend to a higher regional or national level – setting practice and ethical standards and licensure parameters, or gathering research data and evidence so the profession can influence public policy. In any case, an association's success hinges on its contemporary relevance and ability to function effectively, efficiently, and sustainably (CNA 2006b).

Because professional associations function in diverse social, political, and economic environments, monitoring those environments and influencing public policy require sophisticated advocacy skills and sustained investments of time and focus. Associations that identify issues, gather data, and formulate positions and strategies regarding health care systems, health issues, regulation, or professional practice are well-positioned to have a leadership role in forming healthy public policy.

Healthy public policy entails assessments, targets, and measures that support access to health care and promote investments in public health and health systems so skills, resources, and infrastructure meet society's needs. It considers the consequences of public policy for health outcomes (Rains & Barton-Kriese 2001) and expresses concern for health and equity in all areas of policy (WHO 1998). On a global scale, it invests in actions that advance everyone's health.

Advocacy is a core attribute of nurses' professional identity and a major function of associations. While nursing practice and ethical standards guide nursing interventions to help patients attain the highest possible level of health and well-being (CNA 2008), advocacy for policies aimed at safeguarding the rights of patients is also a professional responsibility. The concept of clinical agency (Benner et al. 1996) articulates the extended role of nurses: it goes beyond direct care to include representing patients' interests within the interdisciplinary team and engaging professional associations that work with professionals, key stakeholders, and decision-makers to lobby for policies that protect the public's right to receive care that meets high standards.

Governments are responsible for advancing a public policy framework that guides their action or inaction on political, social, cultural, or economic priorities at the local, national, or international level (CNA 2007b). Analyzing a government's track record on policy issues, forging relationships with decision-makers, and contributing evidence and perspectives are essential to the policy process.

Influencing policy through advocacy can be arduous and time-consuming; it requires considerable planning and endurance. The essential steps in creating a successful policy agenda are defining the preferred outcomes and adopting an implementation strategy. Building alliances to articulate the direction this effort will take lays the foundation for subsequent steps – building evidence, evaluating core values, and engaging public and private stakeholders (Shamian et al. 2006).

Historically, the public's perception of where nurses fit into the health care system, and the fact that most nurses are women, have dampened the profession's voice in the policy arena. However, the increasing number of nurse scientists worldwide and their links with professional associations have created opportunities for the nursing profession to identify policy priorities, bring evidence to the fore, and help translate evidence into public policy options. Establishing an association that has the skills and effectiveness to lead changes in public policy calls for a range of investments:

- An infrastructure with human resources and expertise to support evidence-gathering;
- Consultation with researchers and experts in the field, and with government decision-makers, to define the scope of the issue at hand, build a solid evidence base, and gauge the government's values and perspectives;
- Alliance-building and focused communications with professionals, professional organizations, and public stakeholders that will broaden insights and engender shared values, goals, and overall vision; and
- Persistence in advancing priority issues.

Associations can influence policy in a number of ways, first by gathering and analyzing information that clarifies the nature and scope of a problem, and that sheds light on the policy options as well as on the cost of taking or not taking action (CNA 2006c). To establish its credibility in this process, an association

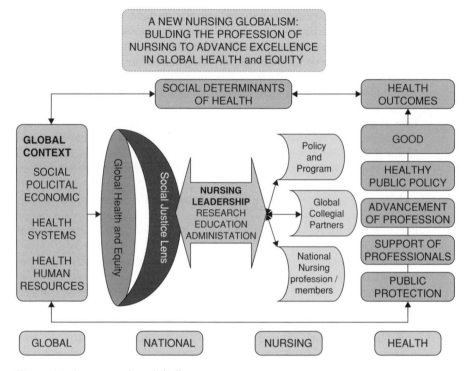

Figure 6.1 A new nursing globalism.

must develop research questions regarding key issues, then review related policies and literature. Consultation with association members, stakeholders, and the public is essential because policy options may need to be adjusted so values and goals are aligned with realities. Targeting important messages to specific vested interests can build and strengthen the network that favors the proposed policy, which in turn leads to further dissemination of key messages and enhances the support base.

An association must engage its members in the policy process and equip them with sound evidence and a rationale. Evidence-based position statements that clarify the association's perspective are a useful mechanism for this purpose. They increase the awareness of members as well as other professional organizations, the public, and government, and align policy positions with the association's goals, values, and beliefs. Figure 6.1 illustrates a process for developing position statements by assimilating evidence and consulting with members, experts, and stakeholders.

Building the profession globally

National associations worldwide have an instrumental role in developing a nursing profession that robustly contributes to health systems and outcomes amid rapid globalization. Although the barriers to forming a credible and sustainable association vary, the successful ones have several things in common. Their leaders build an infrastructure of members that has sufficient resources to make the association relevant to nurses and the community, the association effectively addresses the priorities set by members, and it assesses its impact and ability to evolve and adapt to changing needs.

Over the last century, the profession has built an international architecture under the leadership of the International Council of Nurses. The council, which has a growing membership, is well-positioned to represent nursing's interests on a global scale because it focuses on a wide range of professional, regulatory, and socioeconomic matters. It also leverages technologic advances to communicate and disseminate information. To continue in this capacity, the council must adapt to the shifts in global issues and priorities, shape policy and program agendas, and increase its support for its weaker organizational members, particularly those facing severe inequities.

In some regions of the world, the increasing number of professional groups representing the regulatory, educational, research, practice, and administrative interests of nurses is a considerable achievement. At times, this growth has made it more difficult for the profession to speak collectively. In Canada alone, there are as many as 100 such organizations, with little coordination among them. Competing policy positions and messages have detracted from a focused agenda that otherwise would help strengthen nursing and benefit the public. 'It's difficult enough for nurses to understand these various groups – it's nearly impossible for governments and the public to determine who represents nursing and why it has so many voices,' noted Villeneuve and MacDonald (2006, p. 60).

In a number of low and middle-income countries, the fragmentation or absence of a collective professional voice weakens nursing's ability to advance. These countries bear a disproportionate burden of disease and illness, and their health systems are weak, underfunded, and often lack adequate human resources. Although such problems make it especially difficult to form professional organizations, nursing leaders have nevertheless successfully articulated priorities for advancing the profession.

An increasing number of partnerships to strengthen the profession are forming between nurse associations in developed and developing countries. This enables nurse leaders to leverage their capacity to address both professional and health system priorities. The Canadian Nurses Association, for example, has worked with associations in more than 35 low and middle-income countries for 30-plus years. Its efforts to build capacity are based on the premise that 'strong vibrant professional associations play an important leadership role in the health sector and in the advancement of global health and equity' (CNA 2006a, p. 3). The CNA's International Health Partnership (IHP) program applies the principles of social justice and respect for local ownership in working with organizations on a medium or long-term basis.

Through the IHP, national nurse associations and regional nursing networks identify priorities for ameliorating and perhaps overcoming health challenges. Similar initiatives are under way in the Southern Africa Developing Community (SADC), an alliance of 13 countries, where associations have established the SADC AIDS Network of Nurses and Midwives to respond to HIV/AIDS. The IHP collaborates with participating nurse associations to develop a strategic vision, build technical skills for managing a membership-based organization, and build basic skills such as project planning and budgeting, membership registration, communications with members, and regular environmental scanning.

Box 6.1: Nursing and Health Reform in El Salvador

The fragmented health care system in El Salvador has undergone several changes in the last decade. The most recent change occurred in 2006 when the Legislative Assembly approved the replacement of five health regions with 17 health units in the new Basic Integrated Health Care System. This put clinical nurses in a weak position because, as junior members of multidisciplinary teams, they had less influence than they did as nursing coordinators at the local level, where their visibility was greater.

The National Nursing Association, based on a mandate from its members, worked with researchers to prepare a technical and administrative proposal calling for five regional nursing units to work with the multidisciplinary teams, thereby ensuring the presence of nurses at the local level and high-quality nursing care. Regional nurses and the High Level Nursing Unit, part of the Ministry of Public Health and Social Assistance, endorsed the proposal, which the Ministry of Health approved.

Now, the challenge for regional head nurses and those who work in high-level nursing units is to preserve and strengthen this structure – efforts the National Nursing Association will continue supporting.

The association's success in this case illustrates its capacity to influence health policy. A decisive factor was the involvement of various players and partnerships. Among them was the Canadian Nurses Association, which provided technical support and resources.

Maria Ángela Elías Marroquín
National Nursing Association of El Salvador
University of El Salvador

Reproduced with permission from Maria Ángela Elías Marroquín of National Nursing Association of El Salvador

---

A main IHP function is helping associations and networks build knowledge through self-assessment, priority-setting, strategic planning, and monitoring of results. The Association Capacity Development Framework (CNA 2006a) offers a practical tool that associations can use to evaluate their capacity, orientations, and functions, and to develop, implement, and evaluate a strategic plan.

In El Salvador, the National Nursing Association worked with researchers, nurse leaders, and its members on a strategy to influence health reform (Box 6.1). This strategy has been instrumental in positioning nurse leaders in a new health care system, an achievement due largely to broad consultation and strategic thinking on the part of the association with support from international partners.

Another IHP collaborative effort was a study conducted by the Ethiopian Nurses Association (2008) in five regions to assess occupational health and safety related to needle-stick injuries. It found that 48.1–60.7% of nurses surveyed had sustained such an injury in the previous year. Of these, only 7% reported the incident to managers; the nurses opted instead to respond individually, because of a lack of reporting mechanisms and few protocols. These results prompted the association to examine factors that enabled needle-stick injuries to occur, including institutional and national policies and practices. The outcome has been a capacity-building initiative by the association to support ongoing assessment, education, and advocacy aimed at improving occupational health and safety, particularly regarding needle-stick injuries.

Nurse associations worldwide acknowledge the IHP's contribution in helping them build their leadership and capacity amid very challenging economic, political, and social circumstances. The partnership values and respects autonomy, self-determination, and leadership founded on knowledge and advocacy. It introduces associations to analytical skills and practices that foster their, and the profession's, development based on the best available evidence. Initiatives have helped numerous fledgling associations to articulate and implement their strategic vision, which boosts membership, makes them relevant locally and nationally, and enables many to join the International Council of Nurses and thereby enter the international professional community.

A new nursing globalism

Building professional nursing necessarily involves, and is reflective of, the evolving and diverse social contexts within which nurses are educated, prepared, and deployed. These contexts ultimately influence practice at the bedside, whether the issue is treating an infection caused by a needle-stick injury or caring for a tuberculosis patient or a heroin addict in a safe-injection facility. Social contexts also impact the effectiveness of nursing's influence on policy debates and the degree to which they can exert such influence.

The principles related to global health and equity are at the heart of policy platforms of nurse associations worldwide, many of which subscribe to the Declaration of Alma-Ata (CNA 2002b; Keighley 2006). The principles are in the vision statement of the International Council of Nurses (1999), at the core of much of the council's policy work, and echoed in the values and belief statements of many of its members and other stakeholders. The Global Commission on the Social Determinants of Health, which was to deliver its final report in the fourth quarter of 2008, is likely to assert that equity in health and social justice is the most important consideration for all nations. The report is expected to call for health equity in all policies, thereby reinforcing the central role of health and health equity in social development.

These positions are central to notions of global social responsibility – the collective responsibility to understand and redress global as well as local inequities. Better access to education, greater mobility and connections, and technology that opens the door to knowledge, values, beliefs, and cultural wealth offer numerous benefits. Among these benefits are a greater appreciation of diversity and local obstacles to health, a higher value on nurse well-being, and more awareness of nurses' successes, failures, and risks. Global social responsibility includes reflexivity (Cohen & Kennedy 2000), which for nurses means the imperative to build the profession in a way that enables nurses not only to meet local health needs and shape research, but also proactively to analyze emerging trends and priorities, and integrate evidence and knowledge into innovations that better equip the profession to have a leadership role in health systems.

A new nursing globalism contrasts with aspects of economic globalization that reinforce competition and territoriality. Unlike the drive for individual gain, it seeks to achieve sustainable, locally desired results; is built on mutual respect and careful consideration of contexts, issues, and other factors; and provides resources to build capacity and collegiality, which in turn strengthen nursing leadership and foster the growth of a professional infrastructure – one that responds to the critical needs of health systems and populations.

Conclusions

Many social, political, economic, and professional factors affect nursing as it evolves on the global stage to promote nurse leadership, the profession's relevance, and health care quality. Professionals who observe and investigate emerging issues, build upon evidence-based knowledge, use this knowledge to inform agendas for innovation or change, and work together locally and globally to influence healthy public policy will instill the strength that nursing needs to adapt to diverse and complex challenges worldwide.

A necessary model of inquiry and practice within and between professional associations is one that gathers evidence to support policy advocacy and ensures that nurses' voices are heard. Nurse associations and their members gain strength when they use values and beliefs inherent in a new nursing globalism to leverage the visions and expertise of nursing leaders everywhere through results-oriented partnerships. Forging international partnerships, particularly between associations in developing and developed countries, is a powerful way to enhance a profession that collectively addresses health system needs, health priorities, professional challenges, and inequities.

A new nursing globalism offers nurses an opportunity to bolster their contribution to world health in a manner that is accountable, ethical, and safe, that favors local ownership and autonomy, and that embraces the principles and values of health equity and social justice.

References

Armstrong, P. (1993) Women's health care work: Nursing in context. In P. Armstrong, J. Choiniere, E. Day (Eds) *Vital signs: Nursing in transition.* Toronto: Garamond Press.

Benner, P., Tanner, C. & Chesla, C. (1996) *Expertise in nursing practice: Caring, clinical judgment and ethics.* New York: Springer Publishing.

Bowden, P. (1997) *Caring: Gender-sensitive ethics.* London: Routledge.

Canadian Nurses Association (2002a) *The unique contribution of registered nurses.* Ottawa: Canadian Nurses Association.

Canadian Nurses Association (2002b) *Global health and equity: Position statement.* Ottawa: Canadian Nurses Association.

Canadian Nurses Association (2006a) *Association capacity development manual.* Ottawa: Canadian Nurses Association.

Canadian Nurses Association (2006b) *Social justice: A means to an end, an end in itself.* Ottawa: Canadian Nurses Association.

Canadian Nurses Association (2006c) *Toward 2020: A vision for nursing.* Ottawa: Canadian Nurses Association.

Canadian Nurses Association (2007a) *Canadian regulatory framework for registered nurses.* Ottawa: Canadian Nurses Association.

Canadian Nurses Association (2007b) *Influencing public policy: Strategies and tactics.* Ottawa: Canadian Nurses Association.

Canadian Nurses Association (2008) *Code of ethics for registered nurses.* Ottawa: Canadian Nurses Association.

Clark, J. (2006) 30th anniversary commentary on Henderson V. (1978). The concept of nursing. *Journal of Advanced Nursing* **3**, 113–130.

Cohen, R. & Kennedy, P. (2000) *Global sociology.* New York: Palgrave.

Ethiopian Nurses Association (2008) *Assessment of the prevalence and determinants of needle stick injuries among Ethiopian nurses in five regions.* Addis Ababa: Ethiopian Nurses Association.

Gilligan, C. (1982) *In a different voice.* Cambridge, MA: Harvard University Press.

Gordon, S. (2005) *Nursing against the odds: How health care cost cutting, media stereotypes, and medical hubris undermine nurses and patient care (the culture and politics of health care work).* Ithaca, NY: Cornell University Press.

Hughes, F. (2005) Policy: A practical tool for nurses and nursing. *Journal of Advanced Nursing* **49**(4), 331.

International Council of Nurses (1999) *ICN vision statement.* Geneva: International Council of Nurses.

Keighley, T. (2006) From sickness to health. In S. Nelson, S. Gordon (Eds) *The complexities of care: Nursing reconsidered.* Ithaca, NY: Cornell University Press.

Klein, N. (2007) *The shock doctrine: The rise of disaster capitalism.* New York: Macmillan.

Labonté, R. & Schrecker, T. (2007) Globalization and the social determinants of health: Promoting health equity in global governance (Part 3). *Globalization and Health* **3**, 7.

Marks, S. (1994) *Divided sisterhood: Race, class, and gender in the South African nursing profession.* Johannesburg: Witwatersrand University Press.

Marmot, M. & Wilkinson, R.G. (2006) *Social determinants of health.* Oxford: Oxford University Press.

McCoppin, B. & Gardner, H. (1994) *Tradition and reality: Nursing politics in Australia.* Melbourne: Churchill Livingstone.

Nelson, S. (2006) Ethical expertise and the problem of the good nurse. In S. Nelson & S. Gordon (Eds) *The complexities of care: Nursing reconsidered.* Ithaca, NY: Cornell University Press.

Nelson, S. & Gordon, S. (Eds) (2006) *The complexities of care: Nursing reconsidered.* Ithaca, NY: Cornell University Press.

Nicklin, W. & Stipich, N. (2005) Enhancing skills for evidence-based healthcare leadership: The Executive Training for Research Application (EXTRA) program. *Canadian Journal of Nursing Leadership* **18**(3), 35–44.

Oulton, J. (2006) Inside view. *International Nursing Review* **53**, 170.

Rains, J. & Barton-Kriese, P. (2001) Developing political competence: A comparative study across disciplines. *Public Health Nursing* **18**(4), 219–224.

Raphael, D. (2003) Addressing the social determinants of health in Canada: Bridging the gap between research findings and public policy. Presentation at 'The Social Determinants of Health Across the Life-Span,' Toronto, November 29–December 1.

Registered Nurses' Association of Ontario (2007) *Professionalism in nursing.* Toronto: Registered Nurses' Association of Ontario.

Rispel, L. (1995) Challenges facing nurses in the Republic of South Africa. *Journal of Nursing Scholarship* **27**(3), 231–234.

Rispel, L. & Schneider, H. (1989) Professionalization of South African nursing: Who benefits? In L. Rispel (Ed) *Nursing at the crossroads: Organization, professionalisation, and politicization.* Johannesburg: Center for the Study of Health Policy.

Sachs, J.D. (2001) *Macroeconomics and health: Investing in health for economic development. Report of the Commission on Macroeconomics and Health.* Geneva: World Health Organization.

Shamian, J., Skelton-Green, J. & Villeneuve, M. (2006) Policy: The essential link in successful transformation. In M. McIntyre, E. Thomlinson & C. McDonald (Eds) *Realities of Canadian nursing: Professional, practice, and power issues*, 2nd Edn. Philadelphia: Lippincott Williams & Wilkins.

Shaw, S. (2007) *International Council of Nurses: Nursing leadership.* Oxford: Blackwell.

Sullivan, W. & Benner, P. (2005) Challenges to professionalism: Work integrity and the call to renew and strengthen the social contract of the professions. *American Journal of Critical Care* **14**(1), 78–84.

Villeneuve, M. & MacDonald, J. (2006) *Toward 2020: Visions for nursing.* Ottawa: Canadian Nurses Association.

Webber, J.A. (2001) Fragmented, frustrated, and trapped: Nurses in post-apartheid transition. PhD thesis, University of KwaZulu Natal, South Africa.

Welchman, J. & Griener, G. (2005) Patient advocacy and professional associations: Individual and collective responsibilities. *Nursing Ethics* **12**(3), 296–304.

Witz, A. (1992) *Professions and patriarchy.* London: Routledge.

World Health Organization (1998) *WHO health promotion glossary.* Geneva: WHO.

World Health Organization (2007) *Interim statement of the Commission on Social Determinants of Health 2007.* Geneva: WHO.

Wynd, C. (2003) Current factors contributing to professionalism in nursing. *Journal of Professional Nursing* **19**(5), 251–261.

Chapter 7
Defining the research problem

Junko Tashiro & William L. Holzemer

Identifying problems for research

Nursing research seeks to provide evidence that will increase knowledge about health and well-being, support better nursing care, and enrich nursing education. It focuses on many different subjects, including problems and challenges facing clients (individuals, families, and communities), care providers, and care delivery settings. For example, nurse researchers might study the assessment, treatment, and evaluation of symptoms such as pain, shortness of breath, and fatigue; explore the mechanisms of injury and healing; examine infant–mother bonding and the challenges of exclusive breastfeeding; or, at a systems level, assess the role of safe nurse staffing in hospitals and its effect on patient outcomes.

Regardless, nurse researchers start by identifying a problem – maybe something they observe in clinical practice – or by identifying a gap in the knowledge base for nursing practice. Why is the problem troubling? What is happening? Are different parts of the problem related? What causes it? Identifying a problem and then formulating it as a research question leads to research aims and, perhaps eventually, testable hypotheses.

Researchers sometimes identify problems by exploring patient safety issues in clinical practice. They review data from quality assurance activities and consider if a problem, such as patient falls or skin breakdown, warrants further study. Some conduct a concept analysis (Knafl & Deatrick 2000) as a way to synthesize and clarify a concept. Others, in keeping abreast of current clinical practice, come up with ideas by reading the literature.

This chapter focuses primarily on literature reviews as a way to identify problems for research. It provides a strategy for integrating findings from a literature

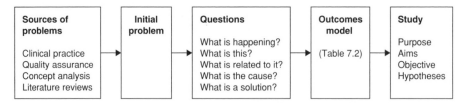

Figure 7.1 Strategies for defining a research problem.

review, observations from clinical practice, quality assurance data, and concept analyses, and for putting these thoughts together in formulating a research problem. Figure 7.1 illustrates the process of moving from the problem source to identifying the purpose and aim of a study.

Sources of problems

Clinical practice observation

If a nurse sees a mother reject her newborn baby or a patient fall and sustain an injury, he or she may wonder why this occurs. Why does one patient survive a procedure when another does not? Why do bench-marking data from a quality assurance program show that patients on a nursing unit stay about half a day longer than those on a comparable medical-surgical unit? Although nurses are very busy delivering care, they must also find time to reflect on their practice to discuss observations and questions with colleagues. Practitioners who share their concerns with nurse scientists can build a powerful bridge to research that leads to high-quality, safe, evidence-based practice for the benefit of patients.

By listening to and observing patients, family members, and other nurses and care providers, nurses learn a great deal about the context and dynamics of care. Often, such knowledge is not shared or formalized, and staff nurses remain silent about things they observe.

Quality assurance data

Health care facilities track procedures, adverse events such as nosocomial infections, nurse turnover, and medication errors, and monitor many other aspects of patient care as part of ongoing quality assurance activities. Depending on a country's legal requirements, collecting quality assurance data may be mandated. As more clinical facilities institute electronic health records, quality assurance will become more systematic and useful for decision-makers.

The key to effective quality assurance is how data are processed, synthesized, presented, and discussed. Many nurses participate in various quality assurance activities – for example, by completing incidence reports, charting patient care in electronic medical records, preparing reports, and, with others, reflecting on data. Bench-marking is a powerful feedback tool, enabling data to be compared with a standard, norms, or expectations.

Nurse researchers in clinical settings often conduct or manage quality assurance because there is a close similarity between the knowledge and skills required for that task and for research. The findings from quality assurance are not research, but rather proprietary data belonging to the institution. Rarely can the findings and the institution's identity be published. Quality assurance has many built-in confidentiality safeguards that are linked very tightly with the confidentiality of patient care.

Research problems identified through quality assurance need to be grounded in a literature review, and the appropriate committee(s) for the protection of human subjects must first approve studies. Usually, a consent form separate from the form that patients sign before undergoing hospital tests and procedures is required before research involving patients can begin.

Concept analysis

Nurse researchers and clinicians are often interested in concepts; familiar ones are pain, medication adherence, anxiety, and depression. Sometimes nurses also are interested in concepts beyond the traditional biomedical model of care – for example, transcendence (recognition and acceptance of the fact that one is dying), mother–child bonding (an existential and perhaps physiologic connection), or caring (nursing actions linked to knowledge and skill, and that support human dignity). Nursing research focuses not only on traditional biomedical constructs, but also on other concepts or phenomena of importance to nursing practice. Knafl and Deatrick (2000) cite various approaches to concept analysis, described in Chinn and Jacobs (1987), Chinn and Kramer (1991), Walker and Avant (1988, 1995), Rodgers (1989), Sartori (1984), and Schwartz-Barcott and Kim (1986). Such analysis helps researchers identify defining attributes or definitions, antecedents, and consequences.

Concept analysis can yield a conceptual framework of key terms, sub-concepts, or concept elements that constitute a research problem. An initial question such as 'Why do some people take their medications as prescribed and others do not?' could become the core concept of a research problem. The process of concept analysis might help the researcher think about patients who adhere well to medication and those who do not. What characteristics differentiate these two groups? The resulting framework may be ready for empirical testing. Such analysis can occur before, during, or after a literature review. It is an ongoing process of reflection and refinement as researchers develop a better understanding of one or more key concepts.

Literature review

Literature reviews vary based on the purpose, scope, depth, breadth, and organization of the material. In the context of evidence-based practice, the term 'systematic review' has been introduced as a rigorous and systematic synthesis of information (Whittemore 2005).

An integrative literature review critiques the methodology and adequacy of theoretical formations (Broome 2000). One definition of such reviews is 'research syntheses that attempt to integrate empirical research for the purpose of creating generalizations' (Cooper & Hedges 1994, p. 5). These reviews are similar to meta-analyses, but they typically are not statistical procedures; rather, they are conceptual analyses that seek to link independent and dependent variables, causes and effects. The author must carefully note the independent and dependent variables, and the empirical evidence linking them together.

A meta-analysis looks at findings from numerous studies involving randomized controlled trials. It integrates the findings to document, with statistical techniques, the estimated effectiveness of an intervention across studies. The statistical techniques explore the respective effect of sample sizes on outcomes. A meta-synthesis, in contrast, synthesizes qualitative research and does not employ statistical analysis (Sandelowski and Barroso 2007).

Conducting a literature review

A literature review gives the reviewer an appreciation of how research and knowledge in a particular field have developed and changed over time. It also sheds light on common research methodologies, instruments, and data analysis methods. Eventually, the level of rigor of both qualitative and quantitative findings comes into focus. The reviewer may read about study results that have yet to be applied to clinical practice, how concepts are defined and measured, and about correlates that, using certain research strategies, may enhance those concepts. Reviews also reveal if other researchers share one's concern about a problem or are investigating the same topic.

The purpose of a literature review often depends on the nature of the question a researcher is asking (Burns & Grove 2005). Reviews in a quantitative framework require a fundamentally different approach than those in a qualitative framework. Quantitative researchers review the literature from the standpoint of how their work will build upon existing knowledge, while qualitative researchers typically conduct a literature review after their study is completed to get a sense of how their findings compare with other results.

A review entails six steps, all of which are important and must be taken at some point, although not necessarily in the order presented below. This is a repetitive process: the researcher constantly returns to the literature to find new articles. The steps are as follow:

(1) Planning the literature review and identifying keywords;
(2) Selecting databases and search engines to locate appropriate articles;
(3) Systematically reading the published literature and, perhaps with a literature review tool, recording what has been reviewed;
(4) Critiquing the research. This entails identifying the strengths of a research design as well as weaknesses that may threaten its validity, and summarizing the major findings;
(5) Synthesizing the literature review, perhaps using the outcomes model described later in this chapter or a more formal meta-analysis or meta-synthesis; and
(6) Writing the review, which presents findings from individual studies and synthesizes the overall results. The review presents the studies' strengths and weaknesses, and identifies topics for future research.

Planning and keywords

Planning involves thinking about information sources that will yield a comprehensive review and identifying keywords that, entered into computerized search engines, will lead to relevant articles. Keywords identify medical conditions, diagnoses, concepts, patient groups, gender, ethnicity, care location, and many other variables.

A good way to find appropriate keywords is to read one or more articles that have been published on the same topic. For best results, the reviewer should work with a librarian on search strategies. Using the right keywords becomes easier with more experience. Initially, they may reflect the reviewer's definition of a problem area. However, because some keywords in databases are based on the biomedical model of care, nursing-related concepts may not be represented.

Selecting databases

Selecting relevant databases is most likely to yield useful results. The first and best place for nurse researchers to begin a literature review is at PubMed,[1] a freely available database at the National Library of Medicine in the USA. Entering a few keywords in the PubMed search engine usually generates a long list of articles, links to abstracts, and the link 'Related articles.' Users can narrow their search by clicking on 'Advanced Search.'

A popular proprietary database in nursing research is the Cumulative Index to Nursing and Allied Health Literature (CINAHL), to which many univer-sities subscribe.[2] The CINAHL software is very versatile and responsive to keyword search terms of great interest to nurse scientists. Another important database is the Cochrane Collaboration,[3] a global effort to conduct systematic reviews of published research, with a focus on meta-analyses. There are many other databases that contain reports, conference proceedings, and published papers. Again, a librarian can help.

To be able to relocate articles and learn which databases and keywords are most fruitful, it is important to document each search, including the name of the database, the search date and strategy, keywords, the number of articles found, and the percentage of relevant articles (Burns & Groves 2005). Software such as ProCite[4] helps manage references.

Retrieving full-text articles online can be expensive without subscriptions to the sources that published them. Entering the exact article title in Google or another large, general-use search engine sometimes leads to the same, freely available article at another location.

Reviewing the literature systematically

Three sequential steps can help a researcher review and critique the literature systematically. The first is to identify the most important variables a proposed study will examine, including co-variates (variables that might be related to the outcome variable), independent variables (interventions), and dependent variables (outcomes). Table 7.1 is an example of how this information might be organized for a hypothetical study exploring the role of massage in pain man-agement. One approach is to read articles focusing on the variables, then to read about the theoretical links between them (Rodgers & Knafl 2000).

The next step is to evaluate how other studies were designed, noting any obvious threats to design validity. Table 7.2 is an example of how one might record this information. The third step is to note the variables these studies

Table 7.1 Example of study variables.

Author/year	Covariates	Independent variable (intervention)	Dependent variable (outcome)
Smith (2000)	Severity of illness Age Gender Type of surgery	Massage (dose, location)	Postoperative pain intensity on ambulation

Table 7.2 Sample strategy for reviewing study designs.

Author/ year	Research design	Diagram					Threats to design validity
			Pre-test	Intervention	Post-test		Random
Smith (2000)	Randomized clinical trial	Experimental group	O	X	O		assignment of subjects to experimental and
		Control group	O		O		control groups?

O, observation.

Table 7.3 Sample strategy for reviewing design instruments.

Author/year	Concept	Instrument	Validity	Reliability	Utility
Smith (2000)	Pain	McGill Pain Questionnaire	Evidence for validity of the scale?	Evidence for reliability of the scale?	Length Scoring Cost Time to complete

measured and characteristics of the instruments used to measure them, including validity, reliability, and utility (Table 7.3).

In critiquing many studies, it is easy to get lost in individual articles and overlook the larger body of work. Over time and with experience, however, good
researchers become experts in conducting literature reviews, critiquing studies,
and synthesizing the findings.

Synthesis and write-up of review findings

Writing a review based on a synthesis of all the information that has been
gathered enables a researcher to formulate a study problem or problem statement grounded in published findings. One can synthesize information by means
of a formal method, such as a meta-analysis or meta-synthesis. Another strategy
is to use the Outcomes Model for Health Care Research (Holzemer & Reilly 1995;

Table 7.4 Formulating a sample research problem using the outcomes model for health care research.

	Inputs (structure)	Processes	Outcomes
Client: patient	• Gender • Age • Education • Socioeconomic status • Marital status • Length of surgery • Pain experience	• Self-care • Family care	• Pain control • Amount of analgesics used • Improved functional status
Care provider: nurse	• Gender • Age • Skill level • Experience with pain management	Nursing intervention to manage postoperative pain	Satisfaction with pain-management skills
Setting: general surgical unit	• Environment • Unit staffing	—	Average length of stay for postoperative patients

Holzemer 2000). Table 7.4 illustrates how the model would apply to research on managing postoperative surgical pain.

The inputs, processes, and outcomes in this model are based on work by Donabedian (1992). Inputs are the client, provider, and setting variables that will be present when an intervention is applied; processes are the client and provider interventions that will take place during the study; and outcomes are the impact of the intervention on the client, provider, and setting.

Conclusions

Nurse scientists identify problems for research based on what they observe in clinical practice, quality assurance data, concept analyses, and literature reviews. This chapter focuses primarily on how investigators review the literature systematically to formulate a well-grounded study question. The steps in a literature review are planning the review, selecting appropriate databases, reading and critiquing studies, synthesizing the review findings, and writing a review. The Outcomes Model for Health Care Research can be a useful way to synthesize review findings and formulate study questions.

Notes

1 www.pubmed.gov
2 Individuals also can subscribe to CINAHL. See www.ebscohost.com/cinahl for more details.
3 www.cochrane.org
4 www.procite.com

References

Broome, E.M. (2000) Integrative literature review for the development of concepts. In B.L. Rodgers & K.A. Knofle (Eds) *Concept development in nursing: Foundations, techniques, and applications*, 2nd Edn. Philadelphia: W.B. Saunders.

Burns, N. & Grove, S.K. (2005) *The practice of nursing research: Conduct, critique, and utilization*, 5th Edn. St. Louis, MO: Elsevier Sanders.

Chinn, P.L. & Jacobs, M.K. (1987) *Theory and nursing: A systematic approach*, 2nd Edn. St. Louis, MO: C.V. Mosby.

Chinn, P.L. & Kramer, M.K. (1991) *Theory and nursing: A systematic approach*, 3rd Edn. St. Louis, MO: C.V. Mosby.

Cooper, H. & Hedges, L.A. (Eds) (1994) *The handbook of research synthesis*. New York: Russell Sage Foundation.

Donabedian, A. (1992) The role of outcomes in quality assessment and assurance. *Quality Review Bulletin* **18**(11), 356–360.

Holzemer, W.L. (2000) Substruction and the outcomes model for health care research. *Kango Kenkyu [Nursing Research]* **10**(15), 360–363.

Holzemer, W.L. & Reilly, C.A. (1995) Variables, variability, and variations research: Implications for medical informatics. *Journal of the American Medical Informatics Association* **2**(3), 183–190.

Knafl, A.K. & Deatrick, A.J. (2000) Knowledge synthesis and concept development in nursing. In B.L. Rodgers & K.A. Knofle (Eds) *Concept development in nursing: Foundations, techniques, and applications*, 2nd Edn. Philadelphia: W.B. Saunders.

Rodgers, L.B. (1989) Concepts, analysis, and development of nursing knowledge: The evolutionary cycle. *Journal of Advanced Nursing* **14**, 330–335.

Rodgers, L.B. & Knafl, A.K. (Eds) (2000) *Concept development in nursing: Foundations, techniques, and applications*, 2nd Edn. Philadelphia: W.B. Saunders.

Sandelowski, M. & Barroso, J. (2007) *Handbook for synthesizing qualitative research*. New York: Springer Publishing.

Sartori, G. (1984) *Social science concepts: A systematic analysis*. Beverly Hills, CA: Sage Publications.

Schwartz-Barcott, D. & Kim, H. (1986) A hybrid model for concept development. In P.L. Chinn (Ed) *Nursing research methodology: Issues and implementation* (pp. 91–101). Rockville, MD: Aspen.

Walker, L.O. & Avant, K.C. (1988) *Strategies for theory construction in nursing*, 2nd Edn. Norwalk, CT: Appleton & Lange.

Walker, L.O. & Avant, K.C. (1995) *Strategies for theory construction in nursing*, 3rd Edn. Norwalk, CT: Appleton & Lange.

Whittemore, R. (2005) Combining evidence in nursing research: Methods and applications. *Nursing Research* **54**(1), 56–62.

Part 3
Quantitative research

Chapter 8
Introduction to quantitative research

Erika Sivarajan Froelicher & Kawkab Shishani

Introduction

There are many excellent textbooks that can help students, faculty, and other scientists learn how to choose an appropriate research design to answer a study question. This chapter does not duplicate that information. Rather, it presents definitions of common types of variables used in research, reviews causality, discusses confounding variables and the essential concepts of randomization, presents two analytical models (parametric and non-parametric), and concludes with strategies for thinking about selecting a particular research design.

A challenge for nursing science novices is that nursing textbooks and articles use different terms for the same concepts, based on authors' scientific training. The challenge is even more complex in the arena of international research collaborations because of cultural, religious, and other differences (DeGeest et al. 2003). Furthermore, an author's education may be in the physical, social, or educational sciences, or in public health, each of which has its own language and conceptual framework.

For that reason, this chapter uses language as in *A Dictionary of Epidemiology* (Last 2001) and other sources (Hill 1965; Susser 1991). Epidemiology is relevant to nursing research because it studies phenomena or disease occurrence and health indicators in human populations. In public health, epidemiology integrates theory, knowledge, and skills in the biomedical and social sciences, and relies on quantitative methods.

Variables

There are three main types of variables in research: independent, dependent, and confounding. An independent variable is an intervention the researcher

Table 8.1 Notation system for variables.

Type of variable	Notation	Examples
Independent (intervention)	X	A nursing care intervention such as a falls prevention protocol or turning patients frequently to reduce bedsores
Dependent (outcome)	Y	A patient safety outcome such as falls, medication errors, knowledge level, or skill in self-injecting insulin
Confounding, or co-variate	Z	Severity of illness is one of the most common confounding variables. Often, it is highly correlated with a research outcome, the dependent variable

manipulates. A dependent variable is the outcome variable; its value 'depends' on the independent variable. Confounding variables, or co-variates, are known to be correlated with the dependent variable and may explain its observed value.

In a study looking at the effect of a patient teaching program, patient teaching is the independent variable, a patient's knowledge of his or her diagnosis is the dependent variable, and his or her education level could be a confounding variable. The investigator may be unsure if the patient's knowledge after teaching is brought about by manipulation of the independent variable or a confounding variable – perhaps knowledge he or she gained before the study began.

Researchers commonly use a notation system to illustrate the three types of variables (Table 8.1).

Principles of causality

Often, the goal of experimental research is to make a statement about a causal relationship. For example, does a change in X (the independent variable, an intervention such as education about the danger of smoking) cause a change in Y (the dependent variable, or smoking cessation). To make causal statements, three conditions must be satisfied: a temporal sequence or the manipulation of the independent variable, evidence showing that the independent and dependent variables are correlated, and control of all other potential confounding variables.

Temporal sequence means the independent variable (X) must precede – or come before the dependent variable (Y) by a sufficient amount of time to be causally related to – the dependent variable. An example would be a researcher who looks at patient charts to determine if the patients were on a falls prevention protocol, then examines incident reports to see if they have fallen. He or she may calculate a correlation between X and Y. However, the investigator cannot state that being on the protocol 'caused' patients not to fall because he or she did not manipulate the protocol in real time and then follow patients over time to see if they fall. Researchers who use this type of cross-sectional study design, in which they gather data from two or more variables at one point in time, can only claim an association between variables rather than causality (Hill 1965; Susser 1991; Last 2001).

The second criterion for making a causal statement – evidence that X and Y are correlated – is often called a dose response. This refers to the quantitative relationship between the dose of a chemical and the severity of the effect it causes.

For example, if smoking is harmful, then smoking three packs of cigarettes is associated, upon analysis, with greater harm than smoking one pack.

The third criterion, control, means the researcher has controlled for all other potential confounding variables (Z variables) that might explain why the dependent variable changed. Of course, it is impossible in any study to control for all potential Z variables. This is why researchers say they have evidence, rather than absolute proof, supporting the claim that X, which they manipulated and which occurred before Y, did in fact cause the change in Y. They are never 100% confident in their conclusion and thus never say, 'I proved that a change in X caused a change in Y.' Instead, they state more conservatively there is evidence that a change in X causes a consistent and predictable change in Y. Researchers sometimes make strong causal statements about their findings based on cross-sectional study designs. In any case, they must consider the totality of evidence before claiming causality (Last 2001).

Randomization

Chapter 9 discusses randomization-related issues in detail – both random selection of subjects from the population to create a sample, and random assignment of subjects to the experimental or control group. Understanding the difference between random sampling and random assignment is critical. These design methods often are used interchangeably or in the wrong context even though they have very different purposes and achieve very different ends.

Random selection (also called random sampling) means every member of a particular population has an equal chance of being included in a study sample. This enables researchers to generalize their findings to the larger population. Random sampling is especially important in survey research, when investigators use questionnaires or interviews to obtain information.

Random assignment (also called random allocation or randomization) means each subject in a randomized controlled trial has an equal chance of being assigned to the experimental or control group. It seeks equal distribution of all known and unknown confounding variables in the experimental and control groups so the groups can be compared without interference by potentially confounding factors. Random assignment requires careful attention to strategies for retaining all participants, as differential drop-out rates among study groups can reintroduce confounding effects (ENRICHD 2000, 2001; Sivarajan Froelicher et al. 2004). It works 'on average,' but is not guaranteed in all instances, as the properties of random assignment apply to large sample sizes and may not be borne out in some small studies. The researcher must identify potentially confounding variables to verify that they are equally distributed among the study groups. Advanced sampling methods such as blocking reduce the potential that a confounding variable will impact study results.

Co-variates: confounding or modifying?

Co-variates work in either of two ways. They may confound the results by introducing bias, or they may modify the outcome or effect. Random assignment seeks to distribute co-variates equally among the experimental and control groups, thus minimizing bias as much as possible. However, the effect an intervention has on an outcome may be different for different groups.

A classic co-variate is gender. By randomly assigning subjects to the experimental and control groups, a researcher can attempt to distribute the percentage of males and females equally. The assumption here is that while gender is known to be related to the outcome variable, gender is not important in understanding how a change in the intervention results in a change in the dependent variable. But what if the amount of change is different for men and women? In a study that tests an intervention such as building self-management skills in newly diagnosed diabetic patients, for example, maybe the outcome is significantly greater among women than it is among men. Random assignment would not detect this potentially modifying effect.

There are strategies for analyzing data in such cases – perhaps, in the above example, by analyzing the data for men and women separately to see if the rate of change in the outcome variable is the same. Although researchers often consider gender to be a confounding variable, it may actually be a modifying variable and not introduce bias into the results. It could generate results that are sufficiently important and interesting to be published separately.

Parametric and non-parametric analytical methods

There are two analytical models that guide researchers when they select study designs, instruments, and the type of data analysis: parametric and non-parametric. Parametric models assume that variables in a study, such as body weight, have been measured with continuous scaling rather than dichotomous 'yes or no' scaling. They also assume that data have a normal distribution – the mean, median, and mode values are equal. Non-parametric models do not make such assumptions. They are more common in public health and epidemiologic studies, in which the dependent variable, such as HIV infection, is often a dichotomous variable.

Statistical tests make this same differentiation. Two common ones, the *t* test and F test, are parametric: they require that data demonstrate a normal distribution. Chi-square and logistic regression analysis, in contrast, are non-parametric: they do not assume a normal distribution. Further training in statistics is necessary to fully understand the implications of these two analytical models.

Research designs

Research seeks to describe and predict relationships among interventions (independent variables), outcomes (dependent variables), and co-variates (confounding variables). Study designs that aim to test the efficacy of an intervention or a procedure are called experimental, those that aim to describe something are called non-experimental, and those that seek to predict something are called estimation problems. Unfortunately, research textbooks use different terms in referring to these designs.

Time, causal relationship, and control group are three important study dimensions that investigators must consider when they select a research design. Can the phenomenon of interest be assessed at one point in time or will subjects need to be followed over time? Usually, the answer is both, which requires a decision about where to begin. For example, an investigator may be interested in postoperative pain immediately after the procedure and on three subsequent occasions. He or she could collect patient data only once (a cross-sectional study) or follow subjects over time and collect data multiple times (a cohort study).

Researchers who apply an intervention and judge its effect on outcomes are seeking a causal relationship. Manipulating the independent variable requires an experimental design, such as a randomized controlled trial (RCT), rather than a non-experimental design.

Finally, will a control group be important – or even possible? If the researcher is simply describing the relationship between severity of illness on admission to the hospital (the independent variable) and length of stay (the dependent variable), then it might not be logical to have a control group. However, control groups make research designs dramatically stronger. Researchers should always consider using control groups because they provide a baseline measure for assessing the intervention. For example, social support data on women living with HIV does not reflect how social support for men with HIV may be different.

Experimental designs

Research is experimental if the design meets three criteria: a manipulated intervention, a control group, and random assignment of subjects to the experimental and control groups (ENRICHD 2000, 2001; Sivarajan Froelicher 1996). The RCT is a type of experimental design that gives researchers the greatest ability to make causal statements (Friedman et al. 1996). A RCT is one form of a prospective trial, in which investigators evaluate the effect of an intervention going forward. It is critical that all prospective studies include a careful plan for follow-up of each subject (Sivarajan Froelicher 1996; Sivarajan Froelicher et al. 1994, 2003).

Initially, the RCT design was most popular in clinical drug trials in which the experimental group received the new medication and the control group received a placebo. However, giving control groups a placebo is undergoing re-examination, as some researchers believe that withholding intervention from these groups is unethical. Today, even clinical drug trials are more likely to test formulary and dose differences than differences between a drug and a placebo. In nursing research, many experimental intervention studies now incorporate 'usual care' control groups instead – subjects who continue receiving the 'usual' interventions for their condition, but not the experimental intervention. Depending on the study, this approach may or may not be justifiable.

RCTs are often single- or double-blinded. Single-blinded means participants do not know if they have been assigned to the experimental or control group. Both groups receive some intervention, but they are unaware of how it differs from the other group's intervention. They also are unaware of the researcher's hypothesis. Given today's demand for very explicit information on the consent forms that study subjects must sign, not telling them which group they are in is less desirable. Double-blinded means that neither the subjects nor the researchers know to which group the participants have been assigned. This approach is much less relevant in studies of interest to nurse scientists.

Investigators who plan to conduct an RCT should be familiar with the wise recommendations in Friedman et al. (1996) and be acquainted with guidelines called Consolidated Standards of Reporting Trials (CONSORT) (Altman et al. 2001). Adhering to these guidelines increases the likelihood of review and publication success.

Data safety monitoring boards have been established to protect subjects from harm in clinical studies (Artinian et al. 2004).

Non-experimental designs

There are four types of non-experimental study designs: cross-sectional, cohort, case–control, and ecologic.

Cross-sectional studies (also called prevalence studies, descriptive studies, or disease frequency surveys) gather data at one point in time or at one collection point. They may be exclusively descriptive. For example, such a study might seek to describe a variable such as the severity of illness of surgical patients on admission to the hospital (co-variate), the frequency of patients' falls among those who are on a falls prevention protocol (naturally occurring intervention), or adherence to medication (dependent variable, or outcome). More typically, cross-sectional studies attempt to find out if there is a relationship between demographic variables (co-variates) and severity of illness (co-variate) or demographic variables (co-variates) with medication adherence (dependent variable). An intervention is not manipulated and there is no control group. Standards called Meta-analysis of Observational Studies in Epidemiology (MOOSE) guide the planning and reporting of cross-sectional research results (Stroup et al. 2000).

In cohort studies, investigators explore how some aspect of a panel or group of subjects, perhaps patients, changes over time (Sivarajan Froelicher et al. 1994; Sivarajan Froelicher 1996). A prospective cohort study follows subjects from the present into the future, while a historic prospective study collects data from medical records or historical documents about the independent variable and, in the future, data about the dependent variable. An example would be evaluating previous data from the ongoing Women's Health Initiative to answer new research questions.

Investigators typically use cohort studies, which do not include a control group nor any direct manipulation of an intervention, to estimate risks. Sometimes these studies examine a naturally occurring intervention, such as an earthquake – for example, a community's use of mental health services before and after an earthquake. They usually seek to describe individual variables and determine if there is an association between the independent and dependent variables over time (Sivarajan Froelicher et al. 1994). A classic cohort study would follow women over the three trimesters of their pregnancy to see how social support, spousal relationships, stress, and anxiety change over time or during pregnancy, or to learn if these independent variables affect pregnancy outcomes.

Case–control studies usually try to determine if an association exists between the independent and dependent variables while controlling for a number of co-variates.

Normally there is no intervention for the investigator to manipulate. For example, a researcher studying drug users might ask, 'Why do some injection drug users become HIV-infected and others do not?' In a case–control design, the investigator might select two groups of subjects: HIV-infected drug users and a control group of users who are not infected. Case–control designs are very popular in epidemiologic studies comparing participants who have been exposed to a disease or condition with a similar sample of unexposed participants. They generate an odds–risk ratio – for example, the risk of contracting tuberculosis based on a comparison of a group that has the disease and a group (control) that does not in a community where tuberculosis is somewhat rare, perhaps occurring in less than 2% of the population.

Finally, ecologic studies examine group rather than individual exposure – for example, to pesticides in the water system. The groups usually reside in a defined geographic area. Typically, such studies are descriptive and correlational, and often do not include a control group. In addition, the data source for the independent variable differs from the source for the dependent variable. An ecologic study might ask, for instance, if public health campaigns about egg consumption successfully reduce cholesterol levels and heart disease in a population. Data about egg consumption (the independent variable) could be obtained from sales records at the National Egg Board and data about cholesterol and heart disease (the dependent variables) from the Centers for Disease Control and Prevention, which, in reporting national statistics, collects mortality data regarding heart disease.

Summary

This chapter reviews the three main types of variables in quantitative research: independent, dependent, and confounding variables, or co-variates. It also explains how manipulated intervention, a control group, and random assignment of subjects to the experimental and control groups are necessary if a researcher seeks to establish a causal relationship between the independent and dependent variables. Co-variates may be confounding (introduce error into the study design) or modifying (alter the outcome or effect). In addition, the chapter discusses the difference between parametric and non-parametric analytical models, which hinges primarily on the statistical assumption about the distributional properties, and briefly introduces experimental and non-experimental research designs.

References

Altman, D.G., Schulz, K.F., Moher, D., Egger, M., Davidoff, F., Elbourne, D., et al. (2001) The revised CONSORT statement for reporting randomized trials: Explanation and elaboration. *Annals of Internal Medicine* **134**(8), 663–694.

Artinian, N.T., Froelicher, E.S. & Van der Wal, J.S. (2004) Data and safety monitoring during randomized controlled trials of nursing interventions. *Nursing Research* **53**(6), 414–418.

DeGeest, S., Dunbar, S., Froelicher, E., Grady, K., Hayman, L., Jaarsma, T., et al. (2003) Building bridges: The American Heart Association-European Society of Cardiology's

International Nursing Collaboration. *European Journal of Cardiovascular Nursing* **2**(4), 251–253.

ENRICHD Investigators (2000) Enhancing recovery in coronary heart disease patients (ENRICHD): Study design and methods. *American Heart Journal* **139**(1 Part 1), 1–9.

ENRICHD Investigators (2001) Enhancing recovery in coronary heart disease patients (ENRICHD) study intervention: Rationale and design. *Psychosomatic Medicine* **63**(5), 747–755.

Friedman, L.M., Furberg, C.D. & DeMets, D.L. (1996) *Fundamentals of clinical trials*, 3rd Edn. New York: Springer.

Hill, A.B. (1965) The environment and disease: Association or causation? *Proceedings of the Royal Society of Medicine* **58**, 295–300.

Last, J.M. (Ed) (2001) *A dictionary of epidemiology*, 4th Edn. New York: Oxford University Press.

Sivarajan Froelicher, E.S. (1996) Tracing myocardial infarction patients for a ten-year follow-up study. *Nursing Research* **45**(6), 341–344.

Sivarajan Froelicher, E.S., Houston Miller, N., Buzaitis, A., Pfenninger, P., Misuraco, A., Jordan, S., et al. (2003) The Enhancing Recovery in Coronary Heart Disease (ENRICHD) Trial: Strategies and techniques to enhance retention of patients with acute myocardial infarction and depression and/or social isolation. *Journal of Cardiovascular and Pulmonary Rehabilitation* **23**(4), 269–280.

Sivarajan Froelicher, E.S., Houston Miller, N., Christopherson, D.J., Martin, K., Parker, K.M., Amonetti, M., et al. (2004) High rates of sustained smoking cessation in women hospitalized with cardiovascular disease: The Women's Initiative for Nonsmoking (WINS). *Circulation* **109**(5), 587–593.

Sivarajan Froelicher, E., Kee, L., Newton, K.M., Lindskog, B. & Livingston, M. (1994) Return to work, sexual activity, and other activities after acute myocardial infarction. *Heart and Lung* **23**(6), 423–435.

Stroup, D.F., Berin, J.A., Morton, J.C., Williamson, G.D., Rennie, D., Moher, D., et al. (2000) Meta-analysis of observational studies in epidemiology: A proposal for reporting. Meta-analysis Of Observational Studies in Epidemiology (MOOSE) group. *Journal of the American Medical Association* **283**(15), 2008–2012.

Susser, M.W. (1991) What is a cause and how do we know one? A grammar for pragmatic epidemiology. *American Journal of Epidemiology* **133**(7), 635–648.

Chapter 9
Sampling

William L. Holzemer

Introduction

In sampling, researchers select a subset of subjects, or elements, from the larger population to study. The subset might comprise people, such as patients; places, such as units in a hospital; or time segments, such as seasons of the year. It may or may not be representative of the population.

The population is all possible subjects – for example, all cancer patients in the USA. There are an infinite number of samples that might be drawn from a population. A sample is a subset of that population, which, in the above example, could be all cancer patients receiving care at a particular hospital. Although researchers use different strategies to select a sample, they are always interested in knowing how representative it is of the population.

This chapter focuses on the various types of sampling and related factors, including sampling error, sample size, sample loss, and random selection of subjects.

Types of sampling

There are two primary strategies for selecting a subset of subjects to study: non-probability sampling and probability sampling (Thompson 2002). Qualitative researchers usually take the non-probability approach because they are not interested in statistically making generalizations about the population (Morse 2000). There are five main techniques in non-probability sampling:

(1) *Convenience*. Subjects are invited to be in the sample in a manner that is convenient both to them and the researcher – for example, by asking patients entering a clinical setting if they would like to participate;
(2) *Purposive*. Subjects are selected conveniently, but with a purpose. The researcher targets individuals with a particular kind of knowledge or experience, such as those who have been in a tragic car accident.

(3) *Quota.* The researcher seeks equal quotas of participant types – for example, of men and women. They are not randomly selected; rather, the investigator invites as many participants as necessary to fill predetermined quotas.

(4) *Volunteers.* A volunteer sample is similar to a convenience sample except that subjects of a certain type, such as people with asthma, respond to an advertisement seeking their participation.

(5) *Snowball.* Like a snowball that grows larger as it rolls downhill, the sample size increases as subjects in a study are encouraged by the researcher to invite others to participate.

Probability strategies, in contrast, seek to ensure that the sample is as representative of the population as possible, thereby ensuring that the research design is externally valid. For example, if the mean age of all cancer patients in the USA is 48.6 years, the sample should also have a mean age very close to 48.6 years. Each time a probability sampling technique is used, it will yield a slightly different mean age. But the closer the overall sample is to being representative of the population regarding variables the researcher is interested in, such as age, gender, ethnicity, socioeconomic background, and severity of illness, the more able he or she is to generalize the findings to that population.

There are four probability sampling techniques:

(1) *Simple random sampling.* Each data element (subject) in the population has an equal chance of being selected. A number is assigned to each person in, for example, a cancer patient population and then the investigator uses a random table of numbers to draw a sample.

(2) *Stratified random sampling.* Each data element in the population has an equal chance of being chosen, but the researcher stratifies the sample based on a certain characteristic, such as gender, to ensure that this characteristic is represented. If an investigator wanted to randomly select nurses for a study, for example, there is a high probability that the sample would be entirely female because, in many clinical settings, all nurses are women. By stratifying the sample based on gender and then conducting a simple random sample within each gender, the researcher would obtain the desired number of male and female nurses.

(3) *Systematic random sampling.* The researcher has a list of names of potential subjects and selects those based on a particular interval, such as every tenth name.

(4) *Cluster sampling.* Sometimes researchers want to sample clusters of subjects first, then individuals within those clusters. For example, an investigator who is studying medical–surgical units in hospitals may notice that patients and nurses are clustered in units. Therefore, the investigator would first make a list of units and draw a sample of them, then take a random sample from within the selected units to achieve the desired number of nurses or patients.

Non-probability and probability sampling strategies yield two main types of samples: homogeneous and heterogeneous. A homogeneous sample might be one in which all participants are women between 45 and 60 years old. The advantage of such a sample is that there are fewer co-variates (variables that may be predictive of the outcome under study) or confounding variables that might impact the results. In the sample of women between 45 and 60 years old, age would not be much of a confounding variable because the researcher has controlled the age range. A heterogeneous sample is one with wide variation in the variables of interest to the researcher, such as gender, age, ethnicity, and level of education. It increases the potential impact of confounding variables on the study results, but it also increases the generalizability of the findings – that is, the external validity of the study design.

Sampling error

Each time a researcher draws a sample of data elements from a population, some level of sampling error is introduced (Hulley et al. 2007). This means the sample is not 100% representative of the population. In Figure 9.1, for example, the mean age in a population of 1000 patients is 36.5 years, but the mean age in the first sample is 34.6 years. A second sample yields a mean of 37.1 years and a third, 36.4 years. Comparing the population and sample means of a variable such as age reveals a potential error in the sampling technique.

There are various ways to minimize such error. The most powerful is probability sampling, in which all data elements in the population have an equal chance of being selected. Another strategy (discussed below) is ensuring that the study has adequate power – an adequately large sample size – to answer the study question. Larger samples have a greater probability of being more similar to the population than do smaller sample sizes.

Estimating sample size

It is important to understand the different strategies available for estimating the appropriate sample size. In qualitative research, which typically relies on interviews to obtain data, saturation means investigators need not interview any more subjects, as the stories that participants are telling begin to repeat earlier stories and textual data have become saturated – in other words, there is no new information. In quantitative research, a more formal mechanism for estimating sample size is power analysis (Polit & Sherman 1990).

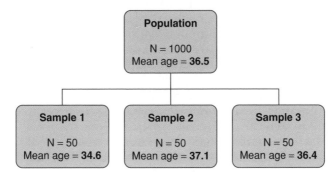

Figure 9.1 Sampling error.

Power analysis is the most precise way to estimate the required sample size, given the number of groups in the design and the number of measurement points. Computer programs that calculate power can be located on the Internet using the keywords 'power analysis software.' Researchers need to understand three concepts regarding estimations of required sample size: power, alfa, and effect size.

Power is the ability to detect a significant difference in the outcome. Researchers calculate a study's power using a complex mathematical formula that is a function of the reported sample size and the selected alfa and effect size (discussed below). To calculate the required sample size, researchers most often use a conventional power value of 0.80.

Alfa is the amount of error a researcher is willing to accept in potentially rejecting the null hypothesis – that there is no difference between the experimental and control group, or the intervention did not work – when in fact the null hypothesis is true. Alfa is typically set at 0.05, which means that 5 times out of 100 (5% of the time), the research may incorrectly reject the null hypothesis when it is actually true. Conversely, it means that 95 times out of 100 (95% of the time), the correct decision will be made.

Effect size is an estimate of how big an effect the intervention had on the outcome measure. One way to think of effect size is as the magnitude of a correlation coefficient – that is, the difference between the mean scores of the experimental and control groups. Ideally, effect sizes are estimated based on statistical findings in the published literature, such as the magnitude of a correlation. In new areas of research, however, this often is not possible, so investigators guess what effect size they think will result from their experiment.

Effect sizes can be small, medium, or large. Some textbooks assign values to these levels. A small effect size (0.20–0.40) is a conservative estimate and requires a larger sample to detect an outcome. A medium effect size (0.40–0.6) estimates a moderate impact of the intervention on the outcome. A large effect size (>0.60) suggests that the intervention will have a very large impact on the outcome and can easily be detected. Significantly fewer subjects are necessary to detect a large effect.

Power analysis is the only statistical way to estimate the required sample size for each group in a study. Researchers should enlist a statistician to help with such analyses. Studies conducted with an inadequate sample size, and thus inadequate power to detect a significant difference in the outcome, are unethical because researchers are wasting subjects' time.

Pragmatic issues can affect the number of subjects to be selected. A quantitative study, for example, needs an adequate number of subjects in both the experimental and control groups, which may be problematic. The investigator needs to determine from the outset how difficult it will be to recruit subjects. If potential participants are extremely vulnerable and recruiting them will be difficult, a research design requiring fewer participants may be more practical. For example, recruiting abused children for a randomized controlled trial could be especially challenging because they are extremely vulnerable and very difficult to contact.

In addition, investigators should consider selecting the most appropriate type of statistical test to analyze data and answer the study question – one that minimizes the need for a large sample size. Many parametric tests, such as the Pearson product-moment correlations test and analysis of variance F, require

Table 9.1 Description of sample loss in a randomized controlled trial (N = 200).

Time	Experimental group	Control group
Baseline	100	100
1 month	96	94
3 months	92	93
6 months	89	90

an assumption that the variables have a normal distribution, which often necessitates larger sample sizes. If a researcher has smaller sample sizes, such as 20 subjects per group, non-parametric tests may be better because they do not include this requirement.

Finally, the time, money, and other resources available for a study sometimes affect the estimated sample size.

Sample loss

Even if a researcher estimates an adequate number of subjects and enrolls them, subjects often drop out over time as a result of circumstances beyond the researcher's control. Some participants may leave the community and others may die. Tracking the number of, and reasons for, drop-outs is particularly important in longitudinal studies so the investigator can present the numbers (as in Table 9.1) and discuss why drop-outs occurred. In this example, the investigator projected enrolling 200 subjects – 100 in the experimental group and 100 in the control group. However, 6 months later, there were 89 subjects left in the experimental group and 90 in the control group.

Differential drop-out rates can lead researchers to draw inappropriate conclusions about their findings. Sample loss or mortality over time also is a threat to the study design's internal validity – the researcher's confidence in the findings. Did the intervention cause the change in the outcome variable or might the differential drop-out rate or some other factor have caused it?

Random selection of subjects

Randomly selecting subjects from a population for a study enhances the external validity, or generalizability, of a research design. Randomly assigning them to either the experimental or control group is not a sampling issue, but rather an issue of reducing threats to the internal validity of the research design by ensuring that subjects in the sample have an equal chance of being in the experimental or control group.

There are two types of randomness:

(1) *Random selection.* Each data element has an equal probability of being selected for inclusion in the study sample. Random selection minimizes threats to the external validity of the findings.
(2) *Random assignment.* Each data element has an equal probability of being assigned to either the experimental or control group. Random assignment

is required in randomized controlled trials. It minimizes threats to the internal validity of the findings.

Summary

This chapter discusses two main sampling techniques: non-probability and probability. Qualitative researchers tend to use non-probability sampling, while quantitative researchers favor probability sampling so they can generate a sample that is the most representative of the population. Important related topics are sampling error and strategies for minimizing it, sample loss, and power analysis, a method for estimating the required sample size for a study. Power analysis gives the researcher confidence that if there is a difference between the experimental and control groups at the end of the study, the difference will be detectable.

References

Hulley, S.B., Cummings, S.R., Browner, W.S., Grady, D. & Newman, T.B. (2007) *Designing clinical research*, 3rd Edn. Philadelphia: Lippincott Williams & Wilkins.
Morse, J.K. (2000) Determining sample size. *Qualitative Health Research* **10**(1), 3–5.
Polit, D.F. & Sherman, R.E. (1990) Statistical power analysis in nursing research. *Nursing Research* **39**(6), 365–369.
Thompson, S.K. (2002) *Sampling*, 2nd Edn. New York: John Wiley & Sons.

Chapter 10
Selecting instruments for research

Julita Sansoni

Introduction

Selecting or developing the right instrument to measure a phenomenon of interest is very important. When possible, researchers choose standardized instruments – those for which there is published evidence of validity, reliability, and utility. They also try to locate instruments that have been used to study a population similar to the one they plan to study and that were administered in the same language.

This chapter describes standardized instruments, which are always preferable in research. In particular, it defines the concepts of validity, reliability, and utility; discusses cultural compatibility issues related to instruments that investigators have used in a different language or culture; discusses the challenges of instrument translation; and explains how to evaluate and select potentially useful instruments. An in-depth discussion of how to construct a new instrument is beyond the scope of this chapter.

Selecting or developing an instrument

Investigators use research instruments to observe, measure, and count phenomena of interest. Before a study begins, they must test the selected instrument on subjects who will participate. A pilot test reveals how long it takes subjects to complete the scale, if they understand the written or verbal instrument, and if they leave some items blank.

There are two types of measurement error: systematic and random. Systematic errors, which often can be controlled by using standardized instruments, arise from faulty measurement methods – for example, giving participants poor instructions. Random errors result from natural, unpredictable variations.

Nothing can be measured perfectly; even when researchers use a highly reliable instrument, there will be some degree of random error. The goal is to minimize measurement errors so the study results reflect the phenomenon of interest as accurately as possible.

If investigators cannot find a suitable instrument, they may need to reconsider the research plan. Another option is to develop a new instrument. However, this very arduous process can take hundreds or even thousands of hours. It involves researching a specific concept (a comprehensive review of the literature is essential), identifying the concept's relevant attributes, and selecting a scale – a response format such as yes/no or a range of choices such as '1 = very good' and '4 = very poor.' A common first step in developing an instrument is to interview participants and collect verbatim words that could be used as instrument items. For instance, respondents would likely reply with certain key words when an interviewer asks, 'Give me an example of when you experienced HIV/AIDS-related stigma.'

Finally, a new instrument must be useful and demonstrate its validity and reliability. By its very nature, an instrument infers that all those who complete it have some degree of the attributes it seeks to measure. If a scale measures anxiety, for example, individuals may be said to be more or less anxious depending on their response. Another instrument may reveal how much or how little social support the participants have and the nature of that support. An instrument the researcher develops must capture such variations, a challenging task.

Standardized instruments

Researchers select an instrument that gives them high confidence it will measure what it is supposed to measure (validity) and produce results that can be trusted (reliability). Information such as the number of items in an instrument, how long it takes to complete, and its potential cost (utility) should be available when a researcher considers the instrument options.

Validity

An instrument has validity when there is empirical evidence that it measures the phenomenon of interest (Polit & Beck 2004). Such evidence is a matter of degree (Burns & Grove 1997); validity is not proven or disproven, but rather supported to a greater or lesser extent.

There are two broad categories of instrument validity: theory-related and criterion-related (Table 10.1). It is important to remember that, in assessing instrument validity, the question is, 'Does this instrument measure what it is supposed to measure?' In assessing design validity (discussed in Chapter 11), the question is, 'Can I trust the results of this study?' In other words, are there threats to the validity of a study's conclusions?

Reliability

In assessing the reliability of an instrument, the researcher asks, 'Can I trust the data?' An instrument is reliable when it measures a phenomenon such as pain

Table 10.1 Types of instrument validity.

Type	Description
Theory-related validity	Overall instrument validity. There is evidence the instrument measures what it is supposed to measure
Face	Respondents are asked if, 'on the face or surface,' the instrument they are completing actually measures what it is supposed to measure. Example: do they agree that items in an anxiety instrument are related to anxiety?
Content	An expert on the phenomenon being measured reviews the instrument and determines if it covers the appropriate content areas
Construct	Refers to factor analysis, a process for examining how items in an instrument relate to each other. It determines whether or not items that are supposed to measure the same thing correlate highly with each other and have a lower correlation with other items
Criterion-related validity	Captures empirical evidence supporting an instrument's validity
Concurrent	Refers to empirical data comparing scores on one established instrument with scores on a new instrument that purports to measure the same phenomenon. Example: a researcher develops a new short instrument with five items to measure anxiety. He or she administers this instrument and another longer, established instrument (50 items) to subjects in hopes of observing a strong positive correlation, which would provide evidence for the concurrent validity of the new instrument
Predictive	The most powerful type of evidence that supports a researcher's confidence in an instrument. Obtained by measuring something in the present. Example: a newborn baby's status using the Apgar scale) with a future event (e.g. failure to thrive). A high correlation between the instrument and a future event provides evidence for the instrument's predictive validity

or anxiety consistently; there is a similar distribution of scores for the sample in different locations and during different time periods. If an investigator plans to use a standardized instrument to study a new population, he or she must re-establish its reliability in the new sample.

Table 10.2 presents the three types of reliability estimates – stability, consistency, and rater agreement – and summarizes the statistical tests used to determine them. Published research provides guidance on what constitutes an adequate level of reliability. Reliability estimates range from 0.0 to 1.0, with 1.0 being a perfect estimate. However, an estimate of 1.0 is never possible because there is always some degree of random error in measurement. Investigators seek estimates of greater than 0.70 for research instruments. They seek estimates of as high as 0.90 when an instrument, such as the Apgar scale for assessing neonatal health, is used for diagnostic purposes or may lead to an intervention.

Table 10.2 Types of instrument reliability and corresponding statistical tests.

Types	Statistical tests
Stability	Test–retest correlation measures stability over time. Administered twice to the same sample, then a correlation between the two sets of scores is calculated. High correlation means high stability over time. Two weeks is often the timeframe for test–retest
Consistency	Cronbach's alfa measures average internal consistency among scale items. Advantage: can be calculated by collecting data at one point in time
Rater agreement	• Inter-rater reliability (using the Cohen's kappa statistic) estimates agreement when two or more raters evaluate the same group of individuals • Intra-rater reliability (using the Scott's pi statistic) estimates agreement when one person rates two or more individuals. Examples: a teacher rates students on their clinical skills; a researcher rates a mother's breastfeeding skill Both tests correct for chance agreement among/within raters

Utility

Instrument utility refers to additional information a researcher would want to know before selecting a particular instrument. Table 10.3 summarizes the dimensions of utility.

Cultural comparability

An instrument developed for one social or cultural group may not be applicable to another group in that culture or in a foreign culture. A tool that measures anxiety, joy, or mothering among people in Italy might be interpreted differently by people in Finland, Spain, or the USA. Even if groups in a society speak the same language – for example, Caucasians, African-Americans, Asians, Latinos, and Native Americans in the USA – their experiences and the meanings they attach to the language, especially health care terms, may be very dissimilar. Furthermore, customs often vary significantly within a culture between countries, such as the Latino culture in Cuba and Colombia. Other factors that may make an instrument suitable in one situation but not another include age and level of education.

Therefore, when selecting a standardized instrument, it is important to know if the instrument has been used in populations similar to the one the investigator wants to study. If not, he or she must pilot test the instrument in the new cohort of subjects and interview them to determine if it has face validity and appears to be measuring the same phenomenon.

Instrument translation

Sometimes, people in two different cultures who speak two different languages can nevertheless understand the concepts in an instrument. If researchers

Table 10.3 Dimensions of instrument utility.

Utility	Description
Length	The number of items in a scale determines how long it will take participants to complete it. If an instrument is too long and complicated, systematic error because of fatigue or boredom might be introduced into the measurement
Scaling	The researcher wants to know how the items in an instrument are scaled, i.e. how do subjects answer the question? Are the answers true/false, yes/no, rated on a 5-point or 10-point scale? Type of scaling is important because it determines how much variation in response the scale will capture
Scoring instructions	Instructions for scoring a standardized instrument should be clear
Cost	Some instruments are copyrighted; researchers must pay a fee to use them
Time to complete	Researchers pilot test instruments to determine how long it will take respondents to complete them. If an instrument requires too much time, respondents may stop completing it; therefore, some data will be missing
Obtrusiveness	Some instruments are obtrusive – they measure sensitive or personal topics, such as alcohol consumption or sexual activities. The more obtrusive an instrument, the greater the likelihood that subjects will not complete it accurately
Sensitivity to change over time	If researchers are trying to demonstrate a change in the outcome variable, they seek instruments that have demonstrated sensitivity to change over time. Some instruments measure stable traits that do not change over time and, therefore, may not be a good choice
Norms	Normative data (similar to normal laboratory values) are available for established standardized instruments, enabling researchers to compare their findings with those of similar samples. Normative data are available for some quality-of-life measures

believe that this is true of the instrument they have selected, it must be translated into the appropriate language.

However, simply translating an instrument word for word is not acceptable. Conducting forward and back translations can be very difficult when cultural differences exist (Frank-Stromborg & Olsen 1997). Research teams should include individuals who are familiar with the customs and lifestyles of the targeted group and who can help translate. A process called decentering ensures that instrument translation produces conceptually and culturally appropriate words. Decentering attempts to balance the two languages so neither dominates.

In anthropology, etic words are universal and emic words are culturally specific – they cannot be easily translated from one language to another. Etic words make for easy forward and back translation, but both etic and emic terms are necessary for an instrument to be understandable and useful. Accounting for etic and emic words in translations is a long and arduous process. Translations also require grammar adjustments so correct words are used correctly.

Thus, researchers must consider both linguistic equivalence and cultural appropriateness when they select an instrument. Many investigators erroneously assume that members of another culture are homogeneous, or they may overlook the possibility that individual members of an immigrant culture adopt the behaviors and attitudes of the dominant culture at different rates. For example, immigrant students often acculturate much faster than their parents do. These and other factors – including environmental influences, such as hours of daylight when the variable being studied is depression – can affect an instrument's cross-cultural accuracy or validity.

Research institutions often have protocols for forward and back translations. Three or four researchers separately translate an instrument and then submit their work to a different group of peers who settle upon a common version. A researcher whose mother tongue is the language into which the instrument was translated and who is unfamiliar with the tool performs the back translation. Then, another group must resolve problems identified during the back translation. Properly translating instruments is expensive and time-consuming.

Assessing available tools

Frank-Stromborg & Olsen (1997) pose a number of questions that investigators should consider when they decide whether or not to use an existing instrument:

- Is the instrument's purpose clear and does it measure the construct identified by the study's purpose?
- Is the conceptual basis of the construct validity appropriate for the investigator's study questions?
- Are study participants similar to the people among whom the instrument was tested?
- Is the instrument's content current and is there a rationale for using items in it? The date the tool was developed may suggest that language and cultures have changed – that the instrument may be outdated and thus have low face validity.
- Is it clear how the instrument should be administered and scored?
- Is the instrument sensitive, reliable, and valid? Does its developer explain how sensitivity, reliability, and validity were established?
- Can study participants understand the instrument's language?
- How feasible is the instrument in terms of cost and the amount of time subjects will need to complete it?

Researchers enhance the quality of a study and the value of its results by deploying the best available standardized instrument to measure the variables of interest. They find appropriate tools by thoroughly reviewing the literature. For worthy candidates, there should be at least one published report describing how the instrument was developed, what it measures, its reliability and validity, and how the tool is scored. The size of the sample on which it was tested is especially important because that affects reliability and validity. In the past, many instruments relied on small test samples (Frank-Stromborg & Olsen 1997).

After an investigator has identified an appropriate instrument, the next step may be to contact its author to ask for permission to use it. Most authors are pleased to grant such requests. Using an instrument protected by copyright laws requires the author's permission, which, for legal reasons, should be obtained in writing and kept on file for 5 years. Authors who grant permission typically want to know what the target population is, the conditions under which the sample will be studied, and other parameters. In addition, they often want a copy of the results for their own files so they can track the manner, purpose, and frequency of the instrument's use. Some charge a fee based on how many copies of the tool the investigator requests.

Summary

Researchers should select standardized instruments that, based on published evidence, have validity, reliability, and utility, which can be assessed using certain statistical tests. Developing a new instrument is arduous, in part because it must demonstrate validity and reliability. Choosing an existing instrument that has been used in a different culture with a different language raises a number of cultural comparability and translation issues. Investigators should ask numerous questions about instruments in deciding which one would be best for their study. Using a copyrighted instrument requires the author's permission.

References

Burns, N. & Grove, S. (1997) *The practice of nursing research: Conduct, critique, and utilization*, 3rd Edn. Philadelphia: W.B. Saunders.

Frank-Stromborg, M. & Olsen, S. (1997) *Instruments for clinical health-care research*, 4th Edn. Boston: Jones and Bartlett.

Polit, D.F. & Beck, C.T. (2004) *Nursing research: Principles and methods*, 7th Edn. London: Lippincott Williams & Wilkins.

Chapter 11
Experimental research designs

John Arudo

Randomized controlled trials

The gold standard of research designs is the randomized controlled trial (RCT). Clinicians and researchers consider evidence from RCTs to be the most rigorous or trustworthy for the purpose of building evidence-based practice guidelines to improve clinical practice.

RCTs are experiments that seek to determine if an intervention causes a change in the outcome variable. To qualify as such, they must include an intervention (independent variable), which the researcher manipulates and exposes to the experimental group; a control group, which is not exposed to the intervention; and randomization, or random assignment of subjects to the experimental or control group. This means that each subject has an equal probability of being in either group (Polit & Beck 2004). The experimental and control groups should be as characteristically similar as possible. In addition, the investigation should be conducted systematically and under identical conditions for both groups to minimize biases that may be introduced as a result of unexplainable random or systematic error (Petrie & Sabin 2000).

Intervention

Many experimental studies are designed to test hypotheses about the effectiveness of an intervention. The researchers want to understand the relationship between their intervention. A hypothesis that research might test would be, 'Does a certain counseling approach regarding anti-retroviral therapy adherence prompt more HIV and AIDS patients to be compliant?' An experiment that studies such a question will only be of value if the researchers can achieve confidence about the causal relationship based on observations under strictly controlled conditions (Polit & Beck 2004).

Manipulation of the independent variable involves doing something to the participants or introducing an experimental treatment or intervention. The researcher administers a treatment or intervention to one group and deliberately withholds it from a comparable, or control, group. Manipulating the independent variable enables the researcher to study its effect on the dependent variable (Polit & Beck 2004). For example, what effect does the frequency of turning a patient – every 2 hours, in normal practice – have on the development of pressure sores, presuming that the lack of turning causes such sores? The researcher can manipulate the turning so that one group of participants receives the intervention and the comparative group does not.

Control group

A control group is essential when designing an RCT because it gives researchers confidence in their findings. For instance, to evaluate the effect of vitamin supplements on children's growth (the dependent variable), researchers might administer supplements (the independent variable) to the experimental group and a placebo to the control group. They could measure growth before and after the intervention to see if there is a difference. To attribute a change to the supplements, an increase in growth would have to be more than the increase one normally expects as children mature. Thus, a change within the normal range could not be attributed to the vitamin supplement; a conclusion that the supplements caused an increase in weight and height would be incorrect.

A more refined study in this case would compare the experimental and control groups to distinguish the effects of maturation (normal growth and development) from the effects of treatment.

Randomization

Randomization ensures a greater likelihood that the two groups will be similar in terms of personal characteristics so researchers can gauge the potential effect of experimental variables (Cohen et al. 2000). The critical element in randomization is the unpredictability of each subsequent assignment of a participant to the intervention or control group. Researchers achieve randomization by using software or a table of random numbers in a statistics textbook – for example, assigning odd numbers to participants in the intervention group and even numbers to those in the control group (Gordis 2004). Using random numbers and explaining in detail how the researchers assigned participants to either group are important so other investigators can later check the quality of the randomization

Table 11.1 Randomized controlled trial (RCT) with experimental and control groups observed at two points in time.

Random assignment →	Experimental group Control group	O_{1exp} O_{1con} Pre-test	X →	O_{2exp} O_{2con} Post-test

O, observation or collection point; X, intervention.

process. To ensure randomness, researchers ideally should not know which participants have been assigned to which group until enrollment is completed.

Table 11.1 illustrates a classic RCT – a two-group, repeated-measures design.

Hypothesis testing

Research questions are usually rewritten as hypothesis statements. There are two major types of hypotheses: null and alternative.

Null hypothesis

A null hypothesis states that there is no difference in the post-test outcome measure between the experimental and control groups. In other words, the difference between them is not significant. Using Table 11.1 as a reference, the null hypothesis could be formulated as $O_{2exp} = O_{2con}$.

The goal of hypothesis testing is to reject the null hypothesis. When a researcher rejects it, he or she is stating that indeed there is a difference between the mean scores for the experimental and control groups. This allows the researcher to consider the alternative hypothesis.

Alternative hypothesis

An alternative hypothesis states that there is a difference in the post-test outcome measure between the experimental and control groups, or $O_{2exp} \neq O_{2con}$. The mean scores for the experimental and control groups are not equal. This is called a non-directional alternative hypothesis. A directional alternative hypothesis, such as $O_{2exp} > O_{2con}$, means that the mean score for the experimental group is greater than the mean score for the control group.

A simple way to test a hypothesis is to conduct an unpaired *t* test of the mean post-test scores of the experimental and control groups to determine if the difference between the scores is brought about by chance or the intervention. If the *t* test is significant, it means there is a difference and therefore the researcher can reject the null hypothesis.

Other research designs

Among the other common types of research designs are single group, control group, and factorial.

Table 11.2 Single group designs.

Type	Schematic	Description
Post-test only	X O	Not a true experimental design because there is no control group. Appropriate for studying the impact of a naturally occurring intervention – for example, the mental health consequences of an earthquake. No pre-test. The design is weak and suffers from all of the threats to design validity
Pre-test/ post-test only	O_1 X O_2	Often used to evaluate continuing education programs. Researcher administers a pre-test and post-test to learners, then attempts to make a causal statement – that because scores at observation point O_2 are significantly higher than those at O_1, teaching intervention X worked. A very dangerous research design because there is no control group; the researcher has no confidence that the change in the dependent variable is caused by the intervention or some other factor. Not a recommended design
Repeated measures	O_1 O_2 O_3	Might be useful for a descriptive study in which subjects are followed over time. For example, a researcher might measure stress and anxiety level of first-time mothers over three trimesters. Can be used to explore change over time, but not to investigate any causal relationship
Repeated measures design with subjects serving as their own control	O_1 X O_2 (X) O_3	Researcher collects baseline data on a single group of subjects (O_1), administers the intervention (X), measures any change (O_2), withdraws the intervention ([X]), and measures again (O_3) to see if mean scores at O_3 have returned to O_1 levels. Might be appropriate for a drug trial: researcher measures patient's blood pressure, administers a drug that reduces blood pressure and determines if reduction occurred, and withdraws medication to see if blood pressure returned to pre-test levels. Design only works when a 'wash-out' period of the intervention can be documented

O, observation or collection point; X, intervention.

Single group

Four common single group designs are post-test only, pre-test/post-test only, repeated measures, and repeated measures with subjects serving as their own control. Table 11.2 summarizes and describes these designs.

Control group

Table 11.3 summarizes and describes five of the many types of control group, or multiple group, designs.

Factorial

Using a 2 × 2 factorial design, Kimura et al. (2007) examined the barriers to influenza vaccination among health care workers at long-term care facilities in

Table 11.3 Control group designs.

Type	Schematic	Description
Two group, pre-test/post-test	O_{1exp} X O_{2exp} O_{1con} O_{2con}	Classic RCT
Post-test only with control	X O_{exp} O_{con}	Used when pre-test of subjects is not advisable or possible. Subjects randomly assigned to experimental or control group, then post-tested
Three group, pre-test/post-test	O_{1exp} X-a O_{2exp} O_{1exp} X-b O_{2exp} O_{1con} O_{2con}	Explores two interventions (X-a, X-b) and has one control group. Subjects randomly assigned to one of the three groups
Two group factorial	O_1 X-a O_2 O_1 X-b O_2	Both experimental groups receive an intervention, perhaps a different dose of a treatment intervention. No control group
Two group cross-over	O_1 X O_2 O_3 O_1 O_2 X O_3	Subjects randomly assigned to either of two experimental groups and pre-tested. Groups get one of two interventions for a period of time and a second measurement is taken. Then the interventions are reversed and a third measurement is taken. No control group

All subjects randomly assigned.

Southern California. A previous survey had revealed two general reasons why workers did not receive the vaccine: because they had misconceptions about influenza and the vaccine, or they did not have access to it. Kimura et al. designed a factorial study to examine these two reasons in greater detail. The two interventions were:

(1) A 'Vaccine Day' to address matters regarding the vaccine's accessibility and to provide free vaccinations; and
(2) An educational campaign to clarify misconceptions about influenza and the vaccine, and to emphasize the dangers of the disease.

The two levels of intervention were whether or not the workers participated in the Vaccine Day and/or educational campaign. There were four study groups: A, the control group, which did not receive any intervention; B, which participated in the educational campaign; C, which participated in Vaccine Day; and D, which participated in both activities. Table 11.4 illustrates the study's design.

In assessing the effect of Vaccine Day, the researchers compared groups A and B with C and D. In assessing the effect of the educational campaign, they

Table 11.4 Kimura et al.'s factorial design.

Participated in Vaccine Day	Participated in educational campaign	
	No	Yes
No	Group A	Group B
Yes	Group C	Group D

compared groups A and C with groups B and D. This approach also enabled them to test the interaction between Vaccine Day and the educational campaign – whether non-participation or participation in Vaccine Day was related to non-participation or participation in the educational campaign. The findings would suggest whether combining Vaccine Day with the educational campaign is more or less effective than each intervention alone. Because a factorial design essentially combines two studies of one population rather than two populations, it makes more efficient use of resources (Petrie & Sabin 2000).

Cross-over

A cross-over, or repeated measure, design is a special type of RCT in which each participant serves as his or her own control. All participants should be pre-tested before they receive any treatment, then reassessed after each intervention (Bowling 2002). In the first period of a two-period cross-over study, the simplest design, participants receive an intervention or no intervention; in the second period, they receive the reverse. The order of intervention or no intervention is randomized (Friedman et al. 1998).

Hoeffer et al. (2006) used a cross-over design to determine if certified nursing assistants (CNAs) who received person-centered training in how to give a shower and a towel bath showed improved caregiving behaviors and felt more prepared and less distressed when they helped nursing home residents. The study included 15 nursing homes randomly assigned to one of two treatment groups, and five nursing homes assigned to each group as controls. CNAs in group 1 first received 6 weeks of person-centered showering training, then 6 weeks of person-centered towel-bath training. CNAs in group 2 received the same kind of training but in reverse order. Those in the control groups learned the usual showering procedures without person-centered training. The researchers collected observational and self-reported data before and after the training sessions.

A cross-over study by Larson et al. (2005) compared the frequency of use of manually operated with touch-free dispensers of sanitizer for hand hygiene. The researchers wanted to control for an order effect – that is, the effect that using a particular type of dispenser first or second might have on the findings. In the study's first phase, staff in the emergency department used the touch-free dispensers and staff in the paediatric intensive care unit used the manual type. In the second phase, the two groups switched to the other type of dispenser.

The cross-over design is advantageous because a smaller sample size is necessary to assess an outcome and there is less variability within participants, who serve as their own controls, than there would be between participants. This approach also helps control for variation between observers (Bowling 2002).

Threats to design validity

There are four types of threats to the validity of research designs that researchers must keep in mind when they read the literature or plan their own study: statistical conclusion validity, putative cause and effect, internal validity, and external validity.

Statistical conclusion validity

Threats to statistical conclusion validity come primarily from two sources. One is study instruments, for which there must be evidence of reliability. If an instrument is not reliable and the researcher uses it to analyze data, significant error could be introduced into the results and lead to incorrect acceptance or rejection of the null hypothesis.

The second threat source is power. A study must have adequate power to detect the size of an effect if one is present in the outcome. A sample size sufficient to answer the study hypothesis is necessary for statistical conclusion validity.

To establish statistical conclusion validity, investigators need to ask: Are the data reliable? Is there sufficient power to detect a significant result?

Putative cause and effect

Threats to the construct validity of the putative (hypothesized) cause and effect relate to evidence provided in the background of a research study about the theoretical link between the intervention and the outcome variables. For example, there is a theoretical relationship between taking medications as prescribed and outcomes such as undetectable viral load or lower blood pressure. Researchers need to provide a strong theoretical rationale for why they expect to see a change in the dependent variable by manipulating the independent variable.

A question to ask is: Is there a theoretical basis for thinking that a change in the independent variable (intervention) would result in a change in the dependent variable (outcome)?

Internal validity

Threats to internal validity are minimized in an RCT because subjects are randomly assigned to the experimental and control groups; confounding variables are equally distributed within them. Without random assignment, there is a strong threat to internal validity. The change observed in the outcome variable might be caused by a priori differences between the two groups, not to the intervention itself.

A question to ask is: Could the change in the dependent variable be explained by something other than the intervention?

External validity

Randomly selecting study subjects minimizes threats to external validity. RCTs must use random selection; otherwise, the results are less generalizable. Researchers who conduct descriptive studies should pay close attention to random selection if they expect to be able to generalize their findings.

A question to ask is: Are the findings true for other people, places, or times?

Summary

Randomized controlled trials are the most powerful way to test hypotheses about the cause–effect relationship between variables. They generate the highest quality evidence and inspire confidence in the findings. However, some researchers believe that controlled experiments are artificial, because of the difficulty of meeting the requirements for randomization and equal treatment of groups. Furthermore, an experimental design may not be able to explain why an intervention produced the observed outcome (Polit & Beck 2004).

Although experimental designs may be superior to observational studies in terms of their ability to test a causal hypothesis, they are also prone to limitations, particularly when applied to real-world situations. Understanding the four threats to the validity of research designs gives investigators more confidence in the trustworthiness of studies they read about and provides a framework for enhancing the rigor of research they conduct.

References

Bowling, A. (2002) *Research methods in health: Investigating health and health services*, 2nd Edn. New York: Open University Press.

Cohen, L., Manion, L. & Morrison, K. (2000) *Research methods in education*, 5th Edn. New York: Routledge Falmer.

Friedman, L.M., Furberg, C.D. & DeMets, D.L. (1998) *Fundamentals of clinical trials*, 3rd Edn. London: Springer.

Gordis, L. (2004) *Epidemiology*, 3rd Edn. Philadelphia: Elsevier Saunders.

Hoeffer, B., Talerico, K.A., Rasin, J., Mitchell, C.M., Stewart, B.J., McKenzie, D., et al. (2006) Assisting cognitively impaired nursing home residents with bathing: Effects of two bathing interventions on caregiving. *Gerontologist* **46**(4), 524–532.

Kimura, A.C., Nguyen, C.N., Higa, J.I., Hurwitz, E.L. & Vugia, D.J. (2007) The effectiveness of Vaccine Day and educational interventions on influenza vaccine coverage among health care workers at long-term care facilities. *Research and Practice* **97**(4), 684–690.

Larson, E.L., Albrecht, S. & O'Keefe, M. (2005) Hand hygiene behavior in a pediatric emergency department and a pediatric intensive care unit: Comparison of use of two dispenser systems. *American Journal of Critical Care* **14**(4), 304–311.

Petrie, A. & Sabin, C. (2000) *Medical statistics at a glance*. London: Blackwell Science.

Polit, D.F. & Beck, C.T. (2004) *Nursing research: Principles and methods*, 7th Edn. London: Lippincot Williams & Wilkins.

Chapter 12
Research critique

Jeanne K. Kemppainen

Introduction

To provide innovative, up-to-date patient care, nurses must incorporate the latest research findings into clinical practice. Finding the most valid and relevant studies, and assessing their quality and usefulness, requires critical appraisal of the literature through systematic review.

This chapter describes a critique process called substruction and illustrates how the process would apply to a recently published study. The chapter also describes a critique model for evaluating related research findings from multiple studies with the aim of identifying nursing care outcomes.

Substruction

One of the most important and basic steps in critically examining a published study is to determine if there is logic and consistency of agreement among its essential elements, including the guiding theory, the methodology, and the plan for data analysis. A study's worthiness and whether one can apply the findings to daily nursing practice depend on its being logical and consistent.

The thought of critically examining the underpinnings of research may seem daunting, especially to a busy practicing nurse who does not routinely read and analyze published studies, but substruction, an efficient and systematic critique process that many seasoned investigators use, can help (Wolf & Heinzer 1999).

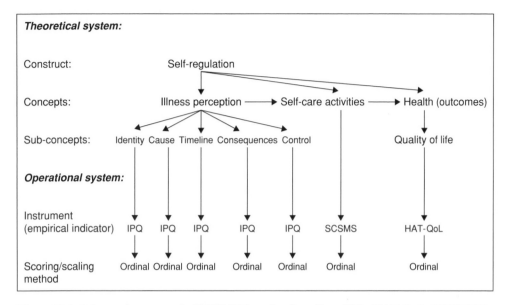

Figure 12.1 Substructing a sample HIV/AIDS study of quality of life. HAT-QoL, HIV/AIDS-Targeted Quality of Life; IPQ, Illness Perception Questionnaire; SCSMS, Self-Care Symptom Management Scale.

Sociologist Jack Gibbs (1972) developed the process, which was later modified for nursing (Hinshaw 1979; Dulock & Holzemer 1991). Simply stated, substruction is the opposite of construction (McQuiston & Campbell 1997). By using a diagram or map illustrating a study's framework (Figure 12.1), substruction enables a reviewer to 'take apart' its structural elements and assess the overall integrity of the design. Often, the links between the theory, methodology, and data analysis are difficult to understand and assess because these elements may be located in several parts of a report or in lengthy explanations or literature citations.

There are three substruction phases: evaluating the theoretical system that guides a study; examining the study's operational system – how components of the theory are translated into observable and measurable phenomena; and identifying links between the theoretical and operational systems. Box 12.1 lists questions that are helpful in substruction.

Evaluating the theoretical system

In a classic paper which applied substruction to the analysis of nursing theory, Hinshaw (1979) cited four, still-useful steps for evaluating the guiding theory. The first step in this phase is to identify and isolate the key elements in the theoretical system, which includes constructs and concepts. Constructs are higher level or more abstract notions that are not directly observable and can be only partially defined (Gibbs 1972). Concepts represent a mental image or symbolize an abstract idea. They include 'quality of life,' 'adherence,' and 'health promotion' (Leihr & Smith 2006). Sub-concepts are the smaller and more specific components of concepts. For example, 'health promotion' comprises the sub-concepts 'exercise,' 'nutrition,' and 'interpersonal relationships.'

Box 12.1: Substruction questions for evaluating published studies

- What is thet conceptual framework or theory used by the study?
- What are the major concepts and constructs and the relationships between them?
- Is the hypothesized relationship between the construct and concepts logical and based on data? What is the evidence?
- Are the concepts and constructs measured with valid and reliable instruments? Do the proposed scores provide data that answers the study hypothesis?
- Are the empirical indicators measured using continuous or dichotomous scaling?
- Were parametric statistics used for continuous data and non-parametric statistics for dichotomous scaling? Is the concept of the normal curve discussed or tested?
- How is the theoretical system and the operational system linked?
- Does the research design provide the strategy to answer the study question(s)?

Source: After Dulock and Holzemer (1991).

The second step in evaluating a theoretical system is to determine if the relationships between constructs and concepts are correlational or causal. If a published study has a diagram of the theoretical model or conceptual framework, the lines and arrows denote such relationships. If there is no diagram, one must search in the narrative for key ideas that make it easier to visualize the theoretical structure.

The third step is to rank constructs and concepts in terms of their level of abstraction, from most to least. Leihr and Smith (2006) suggest a ladder image: a more abstract construct such as self-regulation (the way a person appraises his or her illness or health behaviour) would rank higher on the ladder than a less abstract concept such as self-care.

The last step is to draw a diagram showing constructs, concepts, and sub-concepts and their relationships to better visualize, understand, and trace them (Figure 12.1). After sorting the elements, the most abstract (constructs) are placed horizontally, as a layer, across the top of the diagram; the less abstract (concepts) and least abstract (sub-concepts) are placed below. Finally, arrows drawn between constructs or concepts within or between groups illustrate how the elements relate to each other. Bi-directional arrows indicate a correlational or reciprocal relationship; mono-directional arrows indicate a causal relationship.

Evaluating the operational system

This second phase of substruction seeks to determine if all of the constructs, concepts, and sub-concepts in the theoretical system were successfully translated into specific objective behaviors or verbalizations that can be concretely measured (Dulock & Holzemer 1991). In other words, do they make sense and are they logically and defensibly related to the instrument used to measure them? It is also important to ask if the instrument is valid and reliable, and if it fits with the study's overall purposes (Dulock & Holzemer 1991). Another term for instrument is empirical indicator, or the method for producing evidence about a phenomenon that connects it with concepts or sub-concepts (Marttinen Doordan 1998).

Other considerations are the manner in which researchers measured their data. How did the instrument generate scores or values? Not all studies involve an instrument, such as a scale or questionnaire, that generates data when participants use it. Sometimes researchers administer an experimental intervention – for example, a treatment or patient education program – and then observe participants to see if the intervention had an effect. In this case, does the intervention appropriately reflect the concept or sub-concept in the theoretical system? Also important are how researchers defined their intervention and if they administered it consistently to study subjects (Dulock & Holzemer 1991).

Now the reviewer adds the instrument to the substruction diagram and determines if researchers successfully translated all of the constructs, concepts, and sub-concepts into a reliable and valid measure. In other words, did the instrument truly measure the concepts and sub-concepts in the theoretical system? Mono-directional arrows are drawn from them to the instrument. This enables the reviewer to visualize and trace the connections, and determine if the connections are logical. If they are not clear or there appear to be gaps in the design, the study findings may be questionable.

The last step is to note the instrument's scoring or scaling method.

Identifying relational statements

In the third phase of substruction, the reviewer searches the narrative for relational statements or phrases that clarify the links between theoretical constructs and concepts. Although the substruction diagram does not include relational statements, they are important.

There are three types of statements: axioms, which identify relationships between constructs; propositions, which identify relationships between concepts; and postulates, which identify links between constructs and concepts (Dulock & Holzemer 1991). Typically, relational statements are not labeled as such in a published study, but one can derive them by carefully reading the narrative.

A reviewer needs to keep in mind that few studies are perfect. Even those that appear in peer reviewed journals frequently have flaws in the design and analytical method, which can impact the integrity of findings (Miser 1999). Imperfections highlight the importance of critically assessing published research.

A substruction example

Members of the University of California, San Francisco (UCSF) Nursing Network for HIV/AIDS Research recently conducted a study on how personal beliefs and perceptions about having HIV disease influence self-care activities and health outcomes (Reynolds et al. 2009). Participants were 1217 persons living with HIV disease in the USA, Taiwan, Norway, Puerto Rico, and Colombia.

The following sections describe how a reviewer could evaluate the study using substruction (Figure 12.1).

The theoretical system

The narrative in this study includes a comprehensive overview of the theoretical framework: self-regulation. Self-regulation theory, a highly abstract construct, can help researchers better understand HIV-related self-care activities and direct them to further studies of such activities (Reynolds & Alonzo 1998; Reynolds 2003). It posits that people are active problem-solvers whose behavior is a product of their cognitive processes and emotional responses to an illness.

In evaluating the theoretical system, the first phase of substruction, the narrative reveals the major construct – self-regulation – and three major concepts in the theory: illness representation, self-care activities, and health care outcomes. The propositions, or statements relating these concepts to each other, are evident; according to the narrative, a person's illness representation influences his or her ability to maintain self-care activities, which in turn influence health outcomes. The study clearly defines illness representation as a 'cognitive and emotional processes that individuals use to make sense of an illness experience.'

Three arrows in the diagram from self-regulation down to illness representation, self-care activities, and health illustrate how the construct comprises the concepts. Horizontal arrows from illness representation to self-care activities to health outcomes illustrate the causal relationship between these concepts.

The narrative summary explains that illness representation has five components, or sub-concepts: identity, cause, timeline, consequences, and control, each of which is clearly defined. Identity is the label and nature of the illness, and its link with symptoms; cause is beliefs about the cause of the illness; timeline is the illness's expected duration and course; consequences are perceptions about the short- and long-term effects of the illness; and control is beliefs about the degree to which the illness can be controlled. Arrows in the diagram point down to the instrument used to measure these sub-concepts.

While the text does not explicitly define 'self-care activities,' a definition can be inferred by the way it describes the concept. The text later identifies 'quality of life' as the primary health outcome, which the theoretical narrative does not specifically cite. The causal relationship between health outcome and quality of life is illustrated with a vertical arrow in the diagram.

The operational system

In the second substruction phase, the reviewer traces the link between each concept and sub-concept, examines the instrument used to measure them, and evaluates the methods used to score or scale the instrument. This gives the reviewer a sense of whether the study is consistent overall. It also may reveal a clarity problem or lack of a 'fit' between the elements in the theoretical system and the operational system (McQuiston & Campbell 1997).

The investigators inform readers that they adapted the Illness Perception Questionnaire (IPQ) for an HIV population in order to examine the five sub-concepts in illness representation – identity, cause, timeline, consequences, and control. Researchers developed the IPQ specifically for assessment of these sub-concepts (Weinman et al. 1996; Leventhal et al. 1997). The widely used and reliable questionnaire has five sub-scales, one for each sub-concept. The narrative clearly discusses the scoring method, which is based on a 1–5 ordinal scale.

With the addition of more vertical arrows, the substruction diagram should now begin to reflect logical, appropriate relationships between the construct, concepts, sub-concepts, empirical indicator (the IPQ), and scoring based on the ordinal scale.

The next step is to evaluate the self-care activities concept. According to the text, participants identified six physical and psychologic, HIV-related symptoms that commonly occur and, applying the 1–10 Self-Care Symptom Management scale (Chou et al. 2004), rated the effectiveness of each of the strategies for managing each symptom. The investigators added up the scores and standardized them on a 0–10 scale to assess self-care frequency and effectiveness.[1] A vertical arrow in the diagram shows the clear link between self-care activities, the Self-Care Symptom Management scale, and the scoring method.

The reviewer now looks at how the investigators assessed quality of life, a sub-concept in health outcomes. Their study relied on the HIV/AIDS-Targeted Quality of Life (HAT-QoL) scale, which is valid and widely used (Holmes & Shea 1998, 1999). It measures overall functioning, life satisfaction, health worries, HIV mastery, financial worries, and disclosure of HIV status. On the 5-point scale, participants rated their quality of life for each of these items, from 1 (lower) to 5 (higher). Vertical arrows in the diagram track the relationships between quality of life, the HAT-QoL scale, and the ordinal scaling method.

As a whole, the diagram demonstrates that the researchers used appropriate instruments to measure each of the three theoretical concepts, that the connections between the concepts, sub-concepts, and instruments are logical, and that scaling and scoring methods were clearly discussed. There are no apparent gaps or overlapping ideas in the design.

Relational statements

These are some of the relational statements derived from the narrative:

- 'Individuals are active problem-solvers who experience thoughts and beliefs about having a chronic illness.' This is a postulate, or relational statement linking self-regulation (construct) to illness representation (concept).
- 'Illness representations provide a framework for self-management efforts.' This is a proposition linking the concepts illness representation and self-care activities.
- 'Self-care activities were measured with the Self-Care Symptom Management scale' and 'Quality of life was measured with the HIV/AIDS-Targeted Qualify-of-Life scale.' These are transformational statements linking self-care activities (concept) and quality of life (sub-concept) with the empirical indicator.
- The study posed these research questions, or relational statements: 'What are the illness representations of persons living with HIV?' 'Are the illness representations related to self-care behavior and health outcomes?' 'Does self-care behavior mediate the relationship between illness representations and health outcomes?'

Substruction limitations

Substruction of the above study revealed a congruence between the theoretical and operational systems. Therefore, the reviewer can conclude that the design was proper and that it contributed to the overall validity of the results.

Importantly, however, while substruction promotes an understanding of a study's intent and clarifies the links between a theory, the essential elements in that theory, and measurement tools, it has several limitations. According to Dulock and Holzemer (1991), substruction does not include analysis of instrument reliability, sample size, effect size, or power analysis (a statistical test for determining the appropriate sample size). Nor does it address whether empirical evidence to support the theoretical basis of the study is present or absent. LoBiondo-Wood and Haber (2006) and Miser (1999) discuss these concerns in greater detail.

Nevertheless, substruction has proved to be a highly effective way to analyze a study's framework. It gives nurses more confidence in the integrity of research findings they may incorporate into daily clinical practice.

Outcomes Model for Health Care Research

As nurses become more aware of the benefits of incorporating research into clinical practice, they may want to review evidence from multiple studies rather than just one.

Critiquing the panoply of findings for a specific topic can be challenging, especially given that health and illness research deals with highly complex and multifaceted issues. Studies employ a wide variety of designs with different sets of variables and methods for data analysis, making it difficult to sort out the collective findings. Furthermore, some studies on a health topic may be quantitative and others qualitative. The best way to approach this task is to use a theoretical or conceptual model that brings many factors together into an explanatory framework (Brown 1999).

A good tool for this purpose is the Outcomes Model for Health Care Research, which Holzemer (1994) adapted for nursing, based on the original model by Donabedian (1982). The model helps reviewers systematically organize published studies or variables of interest, sythesize related concepts across studies, and identify gaps in relationships among patient characteristics, health care settings, provider interventions, and patient outcomes (Chou et al. 2004). It also helps them determine what is known or not known about a particular health topic. Researchers have used the model to identify outcomes in primary care (Holzemer 1994) and medical informatics (Holzemer & Reilly 1995).

The Outcomes Model for Health Care Research consists of a 3 × 3 matrix that helps organize variables of interest and points to gaps in knowledge (Table 12.1). It:

Table 12.1 Outcomes Model for Health Care Research.

	Input/Context	Processes	Outcomes
Client			
Provider			
Setting			

Source: Holzemer (1994).

'Focuses on inputs, processes, and outcomes for evaluating quality of care according to the dimensions of client, provider, and setting. Client can include the patient, family caregiver, or community. The term provider can refer to different types of health care professionals. Setting can be a hospital, outpatient clinic, home, or wherever the patient receives health care. A time dimension is incorporated in the horizontal access of inputs, processes, and outcomes that includes pre-event, event, and post-event' (Chou & Holzemer 2004, p. 59).

Researchers can use the model to analyze studies regarding any health care topic. Once completed, the matrix provides an overview of published research. If information is lacking for any of the nine cells, or dimensions, the cell remains blank.

An outcomes model example

Before filling in the matrix, the reviewer should use substruction or a checklist to assess the overall quality and integrity of individual studies. The next step is to categorize studies according to whether they are based on the client, provider, or setting. 'Client' means patients, healthy individuals, families, groups, or communities that seek care because they have a health problem or need periodic assessment. 'Provider' means any health care professional – traditional providers such as nurses as well as non-traditional providers such as folk healers. 'Setting' means any place where care is delivered.

In the following example, a nurse scientist is interested in the relationship between personal beliefs about the causes and meaning of having HIV/AIDS, and adherence to HIV medications. The particular focus is persons living in south-eastern North Carolina, a rural region in the USA. The nurse scientist uses the outcomes model as an organizing framework to better visualize and understand current knowledge regarding this relationship and reviews the literature before conducting a secondary analysis of data from a study conducted by members of the UCSF International HIV/AIDS Nursing Research Network (Kemppainen et al. 2008; Reynolds et al. 2009). In reviewing each published study, the nurse scientist identifies the variables and enters them in the appropriate matrix cell (Table 12.2). Those relating to the characteristics, strengths, and problems of persons living with HIV/AIDS in rural southern states of the USA are entered in the client/input cell. In this case, client/inputs include gender, ethnicity, limited access to transportation, fewer economic resources, lower level of education, coexisting health care disorders such as depression, and the symptom experience of HIV/AIDS. The client/processes dimension comprises patients' beliefs about having HIV/AIDS and the efficacy of HIV medications. The client/outcome dimension is patients' adherence to prescribed HIV therapies. In rural populations, links between personal beliefs regarding HIV medication efficacy and the influence these beliefs had on decisions about taking the drugs are identified.

The nurse scientist's review showed that, despite increasing research on this relationship, most studies involved persons living in metropolitan areas; few examined persons in rural areas. Table 12.2 reflects numerous knowledge gaps regarding HIV medication adherence in rural populations. More specifically, there has been very little research on how the training and experiences of rural health care providers impact rural cultural beliefs that influence health outcomes related

Table 12.2 Outcomes model for personal beliefs and medication adherence in persons living in rural North Carolina.

	Input/Context	Processes	Outcomes
Client	Gender, ethnicity, lower level of education, lack of transportation, health care insurance, rural cultural values, income, coexisting depression or psychiatric illness, spirituality, HIV symptoms, stigma	Personal beliefs about having HIV/AIDS, beliefs about the efficacy of HIV medications	Adherence to prescribed HIV medications
Provider			
Setting	Rural cultural values, racial disparity, rising rates of HIV/AIDS, lack of available specialized AIDS care		

Source: Holzemer (1994).

to adherence to HIV medications. Therefore, in the table, the provider/input dimension remains blank. In addition, there were no studies that specifically tested the effectiveness of adherence interventions related to personal beliefs and none regarding attitudes about the efficacy of HIV therapies delivered by rural health providers, so the provider/processes and provider/outcomes dimensions also remain blank.

Examining the health care setting (third row in the matrix) is important because characteristics of rural health care systems also have a key role in determining outcomes. Factors that figure into setting include available economic resources, organizational factors, and health care delivery methods (Holzemer 1994). In this instance, variables related to health care settings in the rural South include rapidly rising rates of HIV/AIDS, racial disparities, unavailable specialized care for HIV, and the return migration (from urban areas to the rural South) of persons who support those diagnosed with HIV/AIDS. The nurse scientist did not find any studies – for example, about patients who change health care providers, or the availability of HIV treatments – that specifically examined HIV medication adherence in the context of rural health care settings. Consequently, the setting/processes dimension and the setting/outcomes dimension related to provider turnover, patient readmission to the hospital, and morbidity and mortality remain blank. Information was lacking for five of the nine cells, highlighting important areas for future research.

Conclusions

Strategies are available to help nurses and others critique published research, enabling them to identify the most valid and relevant studies. Two useful strategies are substruction (for single studies) and the Outcomes Model for Health Care Research (for multiple studies). Critiquing research should be an integral part of high-quality nursing and an expectation for nurses. Although learning how to perform evaluations takes time and practice, such skills not only enable nurses to find significant study results, but also to apply findings that could have an impact on daily clinical practice.

Note

1 To enable valid comparisons, researchers often use statistical techniques to standardize two or more populations for differences that may exist between them.

References

Brown, S.J. (1999) *Knowledge for health care practice: A guide to using research evidence.* Philadelphia: W.B. Saunders.

Chou, F.Y. & Holzemer, W.L. (2004) Linking HIV/AIDS clients' self-care with outcomes. *Journal of the Association of Nurses in AIDS Care* **15**(4), 58–67.

Chou, F.Y., Holzemer, W.L., Portillo, C.J. & Slaughter, R. (2004) Self-care strategies and sources of information for HIV/AIDS symptom management. *Nursing Research* **53**(5), 332–339.

Donabedian, A. (1982) *Explorations in quality assessment and monitoring: The definition of quality and approaches to its assessment.* Ann Arbor, MI: Health Administration Press.

Dulock, H. & Holzemer, W. (1991) Substruction: Improving the linkage from theory to method. *Nursing Science Quarterly* **4**(2), 83–87.

Gibbs, J. (1972) *Sociological theory construction.* Hinsdale, IL: Dryden Press.

Hinshaw, A. (1979) Problems in doing research. *Western Journal of Nursing Research* **1**(3), 319–324.

Holmes, W.C. & Shea, J.A. (1998) A new HIV/AIDS-targeted quality of life (HAT-QoL) instrument: Development, reliability, and validity. *Medical Care* **36**(2), 138–154.

Holmes, W.C. & Shea, J.A. (1999) Two approaches to measuring quality of life in the HIV/AIDS population: HAT-QoL and MOS-HIV. *Quality of Life Research* **8**(6), 515–527.

Holzemer, W.L. (1994) The impact of nursing care in Latin America and the Caribbean: A focus on outcomes. *Journal of Advanced Nursing* **20**(1), 5–12.

Holzemer, W.L. & Reilly, C.A. (1995) Variables, variability, and variations research: Implications for medical informatics. *Journal of the American Medical Informatics Association* **2**(3), 183–190.

Kemppainen, J., Kim-Godwin, Y.S., Reynolds, N.R. & Spencer, V.S. (2008) Beliefs about HIV disease and medication adherence in persons living with HIV/AIDS in rural southeastern North Carolina. *Journal of the Association of Nurses in AIDS Care* **19**(2), 127–136.

Leihr, P. & Smith, M.J. (2006) Theoretical framework. In G. LoBiondo-Wood & J. Haber (Eds) *Nursing research: Methods, critical appraisal, and utilization*, 6th Edn. St. Louis, MO: Mosby.

Leventhal, H., Benyamini, Y., Brownlee, S., Diefenbach, M., Leventhal, E., Patrick Miller, L., et al. (1997) Illness representations: theoretical foundations. In K.J. Petrie & J.A. Weinman (Eds) *Perceptions of health and illness: current research and applications.* Singapore: Harwood Academic Publishers.

LoBiondo-Wood, G. & Haber, J. (2006) *Nursing research: Methods, critical appraisal, and utilization*, 6th Edn. St. Louis, MO: Mosby.

Marttinen Doordan, A. (1998) *Lippincott's need to know: Research survival guide.* Philadelphia: Lippincott Williams & Wilkins.

McQuiston, C. & Campbell, J. (1997) Theoretical substruction: A guide for theory testing research. *Nursing Science Quarterly* **10**(3), 117–123.

Miser, W.F. (1999) Critical appraisal of the literature. *Journal of the American Board of Family Practitioners* **12**(4), 315–333.

Reynolds, N.R. (2003) The problem of antiretroviral adherence: A self-regulatory model for intervention. *AIDS Care* **15**(1), 117–124.

Reynolds, N.R. & Alonzo, A.A. (1998) HIV informal caregiving: Emergent conflict and growth. *Research in Nursing and Health* **21**(3), 251–260.

Reynolds, N., Sanzero Eller, L., Nicholas, P., Corless, I., Kirksey, K., Hamilton, M.J., et al. (2009) HIV illness representation as a predictor of self-care management and health outcomes: A multi-site, cross-cultural study. *AIDS and Behavior* **13**, 258–267.

Weinman, J., Petrie, K., Moss-Morris, R. & Horne, R. (1996) The Illness Perception Questionnaire: A new method for assessing the cognitive representation of illness. *Psychology and Health* **11**(3), 431–445.

Wolf, Z. & Heinzer, M. (1999) Substruction: Illustrating the connections from research question to analysis. *Journal of Professional Nursing* **15**(1), 33–37.

Chapter 13
Preparing data for analysis

Dean Wantland

Introduction

Analyzing data from a primary or secondary source is easier and much less time-consuming if researchers first plan how they will gather information and then systematically prepare it for evaluation. Everyone acknowledges that raw numerical data sets need to be 'cleaned' for the purpose of accurate analysis, yet few authors explain the data cleaning process. This chapter describes the necessary steps, which include identifying and resolving data problems, and managing, editing, and formating the information. It also describes some common statistical calculations for identifying data problems and how to resolve them.

Good data preparation is essential, but it cannot compensate for a poor research design or missteps in information gathering. Other chapters in this book discuss proper planning of research to avoid difficulties in data analysis.

Developing and storing data

There are many ways to develop a data set. Two simple and widely used software products for direct data entry are Excel spreadsheets and a statistical software package called SPSS, specifically its editor page. Excel and SPSS store data in a flat database, or a table with rows for individual cases and columns for variables. One disadvantage of flat databases is that there are no links between tables. However, for small data sets (up to about 100 variables), Excel and SPSS work well for data storage, manipulation of variables for data cleaning, and analysis preparation. In short, SPSS is a good option for cross-sectional and descriptive studies with a reasonable number of variables. If a researcher is using other analytical packages, such as SAS or STATA, Excel is appropriate; it can save and store files in the formats these packages require. For longitudinal studies in which the same variable(s) will be measured repeatedly over time, a relational database is best.

Developing a code book

A code book lists the names of variables, describes their contents, indicates their type (numeric or character), and, for numeric values, shows the acceptable range – for example, the normal limits for laboratory values. The easiest way to assemble a code book is to use the survey instrument as a template, adding the variable name and acceptable value limits according to the study's inclusion and exclusion criteria. The code book is a useful reference tool as the researcher moves through data cleaning, scoring, and analysis.

Software programs often limit the number and type of characters in variable names, so assigning a descriptive name can be challenging. SPSS, for example, does not allow non-alphabetical characters. An exception is the underscore character, or '_'. A readable name format is four letters followed by the item number. If the instrument is one such as SF 36 Health Related Quality of Life, a questionnaire, the variables could be named SF36_1, SF36_2, and so on up to SF_36. Categorical variables are common in assessments instruments. They often have values of 'never,' 'sometimes,' 'often,' and 'always,' or a variation of such. In the code book, the numeric value of each categorical variable should be listed for reference purposes in data cleaning – for example, 'never = 1,' 'sometimes = 2,' 'often = 3,' and 'always = 4.' Normal lab values and the acceptable ranges for them must be documented in the code book so the researcher can later assess the accuracy of entered data.

The original dataset must be saved before it is manipulated. The revised set is given a new file name and any manipulations should be documented. These steps apply whenever a researcher adds or extracts data from a database.

Missing data

It is not advisable to use numeric values in computer files for missing data, but rather periods ('.'), which make data cleaning and analysis much simpler. Sometimes, depending on a study's scope and design, researchers want to determine the difference between a missing value and a 'no response' answer. The results must be recorded in the code book and, to avoid incorrect findings, later removed from the data analysis when means, standard deviations, or other measures are calculated. To denote missing values and 'no response'/'refused to answer' values in code book entries, investigators typically use '99' and '88,' respectively. In many analyses, whether a participant intentionally or unintentionally omitted a response is irrelevant.

Cleaning data to ascertain accuracy

After data are entered or extracted from a database, and before analysis, researchers need to ascertain the information's accuracy. This means making sure the information was entered or extracted correctly and assessing it for integrity and quality.

All statistical software packages recommend that the syntax (coding) saving function is used for the statistical tests that are run so the tests can be rerun later if needed simply by reusing the syntax file. The syntax files also serve as an auditing function to review for instrument score errors and prior analysis carried out. The time savings that come from saving syntax and reusing it later cannot be stressed enough. Saving and running syntax differs by software package, and it is recommended to review the package procedures for saving and running syntax commands.

All statistical software packages and Excel generate frequency tables – a display showing how often items, numbers, or a range of numbers occur – and the mean, standard deviation, variance, and minimum and maximum values for each variable. Frequency tables can reveal data entry errors. For example, numerical values for gender are usually 'male = 1' and 'female = 2.' A value of 5 in the frequency table would indicate a data entry error and should be replaced with the correct value or denoted as missing. Similarly, an age value below 18 in a study of adults typically would be incorrect. In another study, a systolic blood pressure of 70 would probably indicate an error and necessitate a data review. The researcher should check the code book for normal systolic blood pressure limits and acceptable ranges.

Coding problems are another potential pitfall. For example, if a code is based on gender by diagnosis or gender by symptom, data suggesting that a male was pregnant or a female had prostate difficulties would obviously be wrong. In this case, the researcher could assess the data by using the cross-tabs statistical function in the computer program to select gender and the diagnosis-related group (DRG) code. Another way to assess incorrect coding is to split the data set and select the frequencies statistical function.

Researchers can also assess invalid entries by using the 'if' function in the statistical software. A gender code of '1' (male) and a DRG code of 372, for vaginal delivery with complicating diagnoses, would indicate an error. When such problems arise, the investigator should contact the survey data source and get the correct value, recode the offending value as missing, or delete the case.

Instrument scoring

Most existing instruments for scoring data have been tested and validated. When investigators develop an instrument, the scoring methods should be clear, as tools may be complex. Some instruments require reverse scoring of item values to ensure that all item responses are weighted in the same direction. A higher value means better quality of life or greater depression, for example. Researchers relabel these variables to indicate the reverse values, such that the variable 'cesd_4' would become 'cesd_4r.' To ensure that reversals are performed correctly, the researcher examines the frequencies of reversed variables and their respective original variables.

The next step is to compute the instrument score or sub-scale scores (related to dimensions of one or more variables) according to the scoring methodology.

Researchers often do this by summing the variables representing items in the instrument, using reversed variables when appropriate, and dividing the sum by the number of scale items. This completes data cleaning. However, a number of analytical steps remain before the investigator analyzes the data statistically.

An advantage of using instruments with established validity and reliability is that researchers can statistically determine if the scores and sub-scores they obtained are reliable compared to standard scores for that instrument. Software packages typically include algorithms to assess reliability – that is, whether or not the scores have internal consistency. An important reliability statistic is Cronbach's alfa. Its values range from 0.0 to 1.0. The higher the value, the greater the internal consistency of the scale. Researchers generally consider alfa values of at least 0.70 or higher to be adequate.

Assessing normal distribution

Many common statistical tests assume a normal distribution of data, or bell-shaped curve. If distributions are not normal, researchers can use statistical tests, such as chi square, that do not assume normal distribution. Using frequency tables or graphics functions in statistical software – for example, a stem and leaf plot that shows the shape and distribution of a data set – provides the necessary tabular and visual information to assess distribution. Statistics for skewness (the degree of asymmetry in a distribution) and kurtosis (how scores are concentrated in the center; in the upper and lower tails, or ends; and in the shoulders, or between the center and tails) suggest a non-normal distribution. All of the most common software products include tools to calculate skewness and kurtosis.

Longitudinal intervention studies

Other data-cleaning and preparation issues arise regarding longitudinal studies, or those in which one or more variables are measured repeatedly over time. There are several key elements in these increasingly common studies.

First, the researchers must develop an intervention variable. When they compare a treatment group with a control group, the intervention variable is identified as '1' and the control group as '0.'

Secondly, in most studies, repeatedly measured variables must have a unique name for the initial time period and for each subsequent period so they can be identified consistently. Most statistical calculations, such as analysis of variance, require unique variable names. A common nomenclature is '[variable name]_0' (baseline measure), '[variable name]_1' (1-month follow-up), '[variable name]_2' (2-month follow-up), and so on.

Thirdly, for studies at multiple sites, three variables are necessary: a site identification number, a participant identification number, and a combined site–participant number. The latter helps maintain the integrity of repeated measures data entry over time. Software can generate the combined site–participant number; which is preferable to manual input because it is less likely to lead to data entry errors.

Preliminary data analysis

As we ensure the accuracy of our data set, we begin to determine if the data will allow us to conduct a parametric or non-parametric data analysis. To answer this question, we explore two dimensions of the data, including the level of scaling and the observed distribution of scores.

The scaling of the variables refers to how you capture variation in the phenomenon that you are measuring. Variables such as height and weight are scaled as continuous data with a range of scores possible. Variables such as gender and 'completed high school' are often scored as dichotomous variables because the response is usually Yes or No. Variables with continuous scales capture more variation or variability in the phenomenon we are studying and give us more information than do dichotomous scaled variables.

The second aspect of our data is the distribution of scores to determine if we have achieved a 'normal' distribution. A normal distribution results in a bell-shaped curve when plotted along an axis (Figure 13.1). A normal distribution is defined as a distribution of scores where the mean score equals the median score equals the mode score.

The mean score is the arithmetic average of adding up all the values of the scores and dividing by the number of cases. The median score is the point in the distribution that divides the cases into the top 50% and the bottom 50%. The mode score is the highest occurring value of scores in the distribution. You can see in Figure 13.1 that the mean = mode = median. When this happens, you have met the assumption of a normal curve.

There are two main types of statistical analytical models available which differ based upon the assumptions they make: parametric and non-parametric. Parametric statistics requires that you meet the assumption of having a normal distribution of scores and that the variables in the proposed analysis have been scaled as continuous variables. Parametric statistical tests that are common include tests such as the t or F tests.

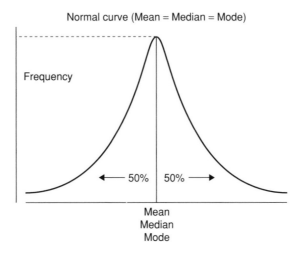

Figure 13.1 Normal distribution.

Table 13.1 Tests of significance.

	Non-parametric	Parametric
Two-groups		
Paired	Wilcoxon Rank	Paired *t* test
Unpaired	Mann–Whitney *U*	Unpaired *t* test
More than two-groups		
Repeated measures	Friedman test	ANOVA
Independent groups	Kruskal–Wallis	Repeated measures ANOVA

When variables are scaled as dichotomous and you do not wish to assume a normal distribution of scores, you choose non-parametric statistics. Common non-parametric statistics includes tests such as chi-square and Mann–Whitney *U* tests. Research scientists from an epidemiologic or public health perspective tend to select non-parametric statistical strategies. Research scientists from the social and behavioral sciences tend to select parametric statistical strategies. There is a comparative parametric and non-parametric test for all common statistical tests (Table 13.1).

For data review purposes, Excel is a useful tool and includes basic statistical frequencies and distribution analysis. The program is generally part of any Microsoft™ package. However, analyzing datasets with a large sample size or a large number of variables, performing advanced statistical analyses, or for projects in which a number of procedures need to be performed is difficult and not recommended in Excel.

There are many excellent statistically focused computer software texts for the most commonly used software packages such as SPSS, STATA, and SAS. These texts describe methods for statistical analysis in the text and are listed by software package in the resources section. These texts can assist you when the time comes to select your statistical procedures and to conduct the statistical analyses. In addition, there are a number of websites that provide background functionality for running a simple statistical analysis. These websites are also included in the resources section for this chapter.

Conclusions

Steps in preparing numerical data for quantitative studies include collection, transcription, management, editing, and formating. Software applications are available to help quantitative researchers develop, store, and later analyze data. An important step in quantitative studies is ascertaining the accuracy of data, which may reveal coding or other problems. A number of computerized statistical tests help investigators assess the reliability of instrument scores, normal distribution of data, and correlation between variables. Researchers are advised to plan sufficient time to clean their data sets prior to conducting the data analysis. Once data accuracy has been assured, researchers must select either a parametric or non-parametric data analytical technique to analysis the data based upon the assumptions required for each respective procedure.

Resources

SPSS

Textbook

Field, A. (2005) *Discovering statistics using SPSS*, 2nd Edn (Introducing Statistical Methods series). London: Sage Publications.

Websites

http://www.ats.ucla.edu/stat/seminars/ (Video clips are available on these sites in using the software but a fast Internet connection is recommended.)
http://www.stat.tamu.edu/spss.php

Excel

Textbook

Chester, T. & Alden, R.H. (1997) *Mastering Excel 97*, 4th Edn. San Francisco: Sybex.

Website

http://library.stanford.edu/services/social_sci_data_soft/docs/software_docs_excel.pdf

SAS

Textbook

DiIorio, F. & Hardy, K.A. (1996) *Quick start to data analysis with SAS* (Statistics Software). Belmont, CA: Wadsworth.

Website

http://www.ats.ucla.edu/stat/sas/notes2/

STATA

Textbook

Rabe-Hesketh, S. & Everitt, B.S. (2007) A handbook of statistical analyses using Stata, 4th Edn. Boca Raton, FL: Chapman & Hall/CRC.

Website

http://www.ats.ucla.edu/stat/stata/notes3/

Part 4
Qualitative research

Chapter 14
Interpretive research methods

Minrie Greeff

Introduction

Nurses often ask questions about the realities they face in health care or a reality they would like to understand better. Such questions may concern nurses' or patients' experiences, the nurse–patient relationship, situations in which patients find themselves, or the context of care and what it means. The need to know is not always related to people in general; more often, it is related to learning about how an individual or group – one with whom a nurse interacts – experiences or makes meaning of something, or about a situation as it exists without any interventions. Qualitative inquiry sheds light on these issues.

'Qualitative inquiry,' 'interpretative research,' and 'qualitative research' often are used interchangeably in the literature. Qualitative inquiry is a blanket designation meaning all forms of social inquiry that rely primarily on qualitative data – in other words, data in the form of words. Qualitative inquiry may broadly mean that the research aims to understand the meaning of human action (Schwandt 2001). 'Qualitative' implies an emphasis on the qualities of entities, processes, and meanings that are not experimentally examined or measured. Qualitative researchers examine the socially constructed nature of reality, the intimate relationship between the researcher and what he or she studies, and the situated nature of the inquiry. They emphasize the value-laden nature of inquiry. They also seek answers to questions about how social experience is created and given meaning (Denzin & Lincoln 2005).

One way to think of qualitative inquiry is as a process similar to building a puzzle: '[Y]ou are putting together a puzzle whose picture you already know. You are constructing a picture that takes shape as you collect and examine the parts' (Bogdan & Biklen 1992, p. 32). Applying this metaphor, Mayan (2001) explained that the border pieces of a puzzle provide clues for building the whole picture. This inductive approach enables ideas or categories to arise from data; the deductive approach, in contrast, imposes an existing framework on data.

Qualitative inquiry entails an in-depth examination of the qualities, characteristics, or properties of a phenomenon to better understand or explain it. The researcher seeks to capture the freedom and natural development of action and representation. Qualitative inquiry does not involve analyzing one or two open-ended comments on a questionnaire or adding quotes or a transcript from an interview without meaningful analysis (Mayan 2001). Rather, by converting data to a 'thick description,' the qualitative researcher gives meaning to the study results. Gilbert Ryle, a 20th century British philosopher, was the first to use this term. Thick description is a coherent account of a phenomenon that provides more than facts and empirical content; it interprets the information in light of other empirical information in the same study (Mayan 2001; Henning 2004). Presenting a thick description that includes ample empirical evidence counteracts the risk of bias (Henning 2004).

Qualitative inquiry methods include:

- Individual interviews, which can be unstructured (to elicit in-depth responses) or semi-structured – that is, based on a set of open-ended questions, or interview protocol, for each participant;
- A focus group interview, which emphasizes interaction among participants. An interviewer asks the group a set of questions;
- Participatory observation; and
- Documents, written anecdotes, audio/video recordings, visual materials such as photographs, field notes, and other materials.

Research questions

The problem a study will focus on guides the types of questions for study participants. The nature of these questions determines the research strategy[1] (Morse 1994), which in turn shapes the questions (Creswell, 2003). The investigator is responsible for understanding the variety of available strategies and for choosing the most appropriate one. Explanatory words in questions specify the emerging strategy (Table 14.1). The link between questions and the selected strategy affects the results obtained and ultimately their usefulness (Morse, 1994). However, the questions might evolve and change during the course of research.

Certain topics or phenomena lend themselves particularly well to qualitative inquiry. Researchers most often use qualitative inquiry to describe a phenomenon about which little is known, to capture meaning (textual data in the form of feeling, behavior, thoughts, insights, and actions, instead of numerical

Table 14.1 Research questions and matching strategies.

Type of research question	Strategy	Explanatory words that reflect this strategy
• Process questions – experience over time or changes, stages, or phases • Questions about experiencing a phenomenon that is a process	**Grounded theory**	• '. . . to discover . . .' • 'What are the processes . . . ?' • '. . . to understand the phases . . .'
• Questions about past events or experiences	**Historical research**	• 'How was it in [time, place, or a situation] . . . ?' • '. . . to understand [a person] . . .' • '. . . better within [a specific timeframe] . . .'
• Questions that yield a better understanding of one or more cases	**Case study research**	• 'In what ways . . . ?' • 'Did the therapy . . . ?' • 'What are typical . . . ?' • 'How effective . . . ?' • 'What is the nature of the relationship between . . . ?' • '. . . is the fact that [something] affects [something else] . . . ?'
• Descriptive questions – about values, beliefs, or cultural practices • Questions about the nature of a phenomenon • Questions about why people in a group do what they do	**Ethnography**	• '. . . seek to understand . . .' • 'How do . . . ?' • 'What are the beliefs and practices . . . ?'
• Questions about meaning, to elicit the essences of experiences • Questions about the meaning of a phenomenon	**Phenomenology**	• 'Describe the experience . . .' • 'What is the meaning of . . . ?' • 'What was your experience . . . ?'
• Questions that reflect interest, concerns, frustrations, or puzzles on multiple levels about a community practice	**Participatory action research**	• 'How can the community become part of . . . ?' • 'What can . . . ?' • 'What does it mean to be in [a specific situation] . . . ?'

data), or to describe a process rather than an outcome (Mayan 2001). This strategy is appropriate if an investigator wants more details and a thick description of people's experiences; it can reveal the story or meaning behind numerical data in a quantitative inquiry (Mayan 2001).

Questions should be as broad as possible rather than narrow, as narrowness detracts from a whole-picture view (Morse 1994). It usually helps to test the appropriateness and applicability of questions on one or more participants before data-gathering begins to see if they are posed in a way that will elicit the desired information. Language and literacy are key considerations when formulating in-depth questions for interview purposes.

Strategies

The appropriate strategy for qualitative inquiry depends on the research question; it will have a dramatic influence on procedures (Creswell 2003). The literature describes a number of different strategies, including narrative, phenomenology, ethnography, case study, and grounded theory (Creswell 2003); case study, ethnography, phenomenology, grounded theory, historical research, action research, and clinical research (Denzin & Lincoln 2005); and phenomenology, ethnography, grounded theory, focus groups, and historical research (Morse & Field 1995). This chapter addresses grounded theory, historical research, case study research, ethnography, phenomenology, hermeneutics, and participatory action research.

Perspectives on qualitative strategies vary and include post-modern, ideological, and philosophical viewpoints (Cresswell 2003).

Grounded theory

Grounded theory is theory grounded in data. Rather than proposing a theory and then testing it, grounded theorists first collect data and then develop a theory based on their findings. Sociologists Barney Glaser and Anselm Strauss, who formulated grounded theory in 1967, believed that theories must be 'induced' from the data: 'Only in this way will the theory be closely related to the daily realities' (Glaser & Strauss 1967, p. 239). The theory evolves during research through a continuous interplay between analysis and data collection (Strauss & Corbin 1994; Mayan 2001). Grounded theory strategies are best suited for studies that examine a process or an experience over time through various stages (Morse 1994).

Researchers use a set of flexible analytical guidelines to focus their collection of qualitative data and build inductive, middle-range theories through successive levels of data analysis and conceptual development (Charmaz 2005). Specific, refined, and rigorous procedures lead to formal, substantive theories of social phenomena. This approach employs deduction as well as induction and verification. Data generate insights, hypotheses, and questions, and as tentative answers arise, researchers construct theoretical concepts and verify them through further data gathering. They sample additional populations, incidents, events, or activities. Participants are selected based on their knowledge of the topic and the needs of the developing theory (Morse & Field 1995; Schwandt 2001). Data comes from unstructured interviews and observation, and from sources such as documents, creative writing, newspapers, and diaries (Morse & Field 1995; Mayan 2001).

Historical research

Historical research, which is chronologic and focuses on a specific time period, examines the interpretation and narration of past events. Most qualitative studies, in contrast, examine current or ongoing events (Morse & Field 1995). Historical researchers in the positivistic or neo-positivistic school try to reduce history to universal laws, while those in the idealistic school interpret intuition and experience. The latter use broad analytical frameworks to study, for example, a great person (Morse & Field 1995). As in all other kinds of qualitative research, the type of data historical researchers collect depends on the question they seek to answer and the information available to them. In addition, they must be knowledgeable about the historical period of their study topic (Tuchman 1994).

Data sources include documents, records, eyewitness accounts, and oral histories (Morse & Field 1995). Documentary and oral histories require corroborative data from several sources, and both inductive and deductive analysis. Researchers' first task is to collect background information, including names, dates, and key events, and information regarding controversies among historians about whether, how, and why these factors are important. Related issues are the reliability of information sources and the investigator's ability to discern patterns (Tuchman 1994).

Importantly, historical research is an interpretive enterprise (Tuchman 1994; Morse & Field 1995). The context of the information a researcher gathers makes his or her interpretation unique.

Case study research

A case study is an exploration or in-depth analysis of a 'bounded system' (that is, bounded by time and/or place), of a single case, or of multiple cases over a period of time (Creswell 1998, p. 61). A simple case study would be one that examines a patient's medical condition. A complex case study might examine the manner in which health professionals facilitate care.

Understanding a case usually requires an extensive evaluation of how things are done. Although a case study comprises both the method and the product of the inquiry (Stake 2005), it should focus primarily on the case itself, be it a person, process, or something else. In 1984, Lawrence Stenhouse, a British educational thinker, advocated the term 'case record' to describe the final product (Stake 2005, p. 445).

Researcher Robert Yin argues that a case study strategy is preferable when an inquiry seeks to answer 'how' or 'why' questions, the investigator has little control over events he or she is studying, the object of study is a contemporary phenomenon in a real-life context, the boundaries between the phenomenon and its context are not clear, or multiple sources of evidence are desirable (Schwandt 2001). According to researcher Robert Stake, the foremost goal is to generate knowledge (Schwandt 2001). He says that while such studies seek to discern and understand the issues intrinsic to a case, researchers may choose to examine cases they believe will ultimately shed light on a problem, issue, or concept.

A case study has some form of conceptual structure and is organized around a small number of research questions that target issues or themes – for example, 'In what ways . . . ?' or 'Did the addiction therapy . . . ?' Such issues involve complex, situated, problematic relationships (Stake 2005). Before the researcher commits to conducting a case study, he or she gathers background information and becomes familiar with other relevant cases.

A data-gathering plan defines the case, includes a list of research questions, identifies research assistants and data sources, allocates time for the study, cites the anticipated expenses, and indicates how the results will be reported (Stake 1995). The researcher explores and describes a case through detailed and in-depth collection of data from multiple sources; the data are rich in context. Sources may include interviews, documents, observation, or archival records. The product of this effort is an in-depth description of a case or cases (De Vos et al. 2005).

The aim of an intrinsic case study is to provide a better understanding of one or more cases. An instrumental case study elaborates on a theory or seeks a better understanding of a social issue. A collective case study furthers the understanding of a social issue or population; it is an instrumental study of several cases (Mark 1996; Stake 2005).

According to sociologist Samuel Stouffer, researchers look for what is common and uncommon about a case, but typically they focus more on the uncommon (Stake 2005). They simultaneously study the nature of the case, particularly its activity and functioning; its history; the physical setting; related contexts (economical, political, legal, and esthetic); related cases; and individuals who have relevant information. In studying a complex case, a strategic decision is when to halt further data collection.

Analysis is a matter of finding meaning in first impressions and interpreting the data. People who are the focus of a case study review rough drafts of the investigators' report for accuracy and palatability (Stake 1995). The final report should be a well-organized synthesis.

Ethnography

In the late 19th century, anthropologists developed ethnography and participatory observation to study 'other' cultures, or, as they often referred to them, 'primitive' or 'tribal' communities (Morse & Field 1995; Potter 1996; Mayan 2001, p. 8). Ethnography has changed considerably since then, but many of its basic tenets still apply (Mayan 2001).

Ethnography, in the anthropologic tradition, is the process and product of describing and interpreting cultural behavior (Schwandt 2001). Ethnographers immerse themselves in a group setting to learn about the group's culture. They develop concepts and seek to understand human behaviors from the insider's point of view. Such researchers learn about people by learning from them (Morse & Field 1995; Wolcott 1999; Roper & Shapira 2000; Mayan 2001).

Like several other kinds of qualitative inquiries, ethnography emphasizes first-hand field study. However, it does not focus on field work exclusively; rather, it unites process and product, field work, and written text. Researchers generally agree that culture is not visible or tangible; rather, it is constructed through ethnographic writing. Hence, understanding what it means to 'write' culture is a critical concern in ethnography (Schwandt 2001, p. 80). In addition to foreign cultures, ethnographers also study specific groups of people in health care, business, organizations, sub-cultures, or ethnic populations (Mayan 2001).

Participatory observation can yield information that is otherwise unavailable. The researcher gains awareness by becoming acquainted with people. The challenge is to immerse oneself sufficiently to understand a group, but not so deeply that the objectivity necessary to record and analyze observations is lost. In ethnographic research, there are four general roles:

(1) The complete observer, who does not take part in the activities he or she studies;

(2) The observer-as-participant, who takes part and the reason for doing so is clear;
(3) The participant-as-observer, who becomes the instrument for data collection and analyzes the data in terms of personal experience; and
(4) The complete participant, who takes part, but his or her purpose and identity are not revealed, which is rare today (Bernard 1988; Mayan 2001).

A more recent modification of the participant-as-observer role is 'observation of participation' (autoethnography), wherein the researcher reflects on and critically engages with his or her own participation in a culture. Autoethnographers attempt to bridge the gap between the public and private realms. For them, closeness, subjectivity, and engagement are more important than distance, objectivity, and neutrality (Tedlock 2005).

In addition to observing, ethnographers conduct interviews – individual or group, formal or informal – and take field notes (Atkinson & Hammersley 1998; Roper & Shapira 2000). Field notes are ongoing descriptions of observed events and people; conversations with and among people; the researcher's interpretations, analysis, and thoughts about further questions to investigate; and personal feelings about the experience (Roper & Shapira 2000). Data sources may include video, documents and records, diaries, poetry, art, or significant cultural artifacts (Morse 1994; Roper & Shapira 2000).

Finding and gaining access to key informants is important in ethnography. Researchers must develop rapport with informants, become comfortable with the setting, and familiarize themselves with customs and nuances of language. To obtain relevant and adequate data, they also must establish credibility and trust (Morse & Field 1995; Roper & Shapira 2000). Ideally, ethnographic analysis moves beyond description to reveal or explain aspects of social patterns or observed conduct. Thick description in ethnography is an interpretive science that searches for meaning within cultural norms, a culturally patterned behaviour, and the cultural context (Morse & Field 1995).

Phenomenology

German philosopher Edmund Husserl introduced transcendental phenomenology in the late 19th century because he believed that the scientific method, while appropriate for studying physical phenomena, was inappropriate for studying human thoughts and action (Bernard 2000). Transcendental phenomenology is not a single, unified, philosophical viewpoint. It includes the philosophies of French existentialists Maurice Merleau-Ponty and Jean-Paul Sartre, and the hermeneutic phenomenology of the German philosopher Martin Heidegger (Schwandt 2001). Several transcendental phenomenology schools have emerged – based on the work of Adrian Van Kaam, Paul Colaizzi, and Amedeo Giorgi, among others – in which phenomenology is both a philosophy and a method (Morse & Field 1995). The two major variants of phenomenology that manifest in contemporary qualitative strategies are hermeneutic and existential (Schwandt 2001).

Phenomenology's goal is not to generate theories or models, or to provide general explanations, but rather to carefully describe ordinary conscious experience of everyday life. Experience includes perceptions, beliefs, memories, decisions, feelings, judgments, evaluations, and everything related to bodily action. Phenomenologic descriptions are possible only by examining the meaning of things – by looking not at what is, but at the nature of what is. Phenomenology accepts experience as it exists in the individual's consciousness (Morse & Field 1995; Van Manen 1997; Mayan 2001; Schwandt 2001).

Descriptive phenomenologists attempt to bracket – that is, identify and suspend their preconceived beliefs and opinions about the phenomenon under study – before they collect data. During interviews, they have no presuppositions. Interpretive phenomenologists, in contrast, do not bracket. In both descriptive and interpretive interviews, research questions 'flow with a clue-and-clue-taking process' (Morse & Field 1995, p. 152). There are seven steps in gleaning the essence of a phenomenon: intuiting, analyzing, describing the phenomenon, watching modes of appearing (present, past, and future), exploring the phenomenon in consciousness, suspending belief, and interpreting concealed meaning. The end product is a thick description of the meaning or essence of the phenomenon (Morse 1994; Morse & Field 1995; Schwandt 2001).

Phenomenology in qualitative inquiry reflects a subjective, existentialist, and non-critical emphasis. It aims to identify and describe the subjective experiences of respondents. This involves studying everyday experience from the respondent's point of view and shuns critical evaluation of forms of social life (Schwandt 2001). In-depth conversations may generate data. The primary data source is individuals' life-world, but researchers may also tap literature, poetry, or art to understand the essence of phenomena. Other sources for gaining insight into human experience include interviews, diaries, and journals. Validity rests in the richness of the discussion. Phenomenologic writing is open to various interpretations, depending on the reader's experience (Morse & Field 1995).

Hermeneutics

Hermeneutics generally refers to the art, theory, and philosophy of interpreting the meaning of an object, such as a text, a work of art, social action, or what a speaker says. Researchers in this tradition study how people interpret their lives and make meaning of the experience (Cohen et al. 2000).

In nursing research, hermeneutics is more often linked to Heideggerian phenomenology. The German philosopher Friedrich Schleiermacher (1768–1834) is generally recognized as the creator of modern hermeneutics, which has several variants. People who further developed this research strategy include Heidegger (1889–1976); Wilhelm Dilthey (1833–1911), a German psychologist, historian, and sociologist; and Jürgen Habermas, a contemporary German philosopher (Schwandt 2001). Husserl and Dilthey were interested in learning about or understanding the structure of human experience. Heidegger expanded this definition of hermeneutics to encompass attempts to understand phenomena as they are presented, how people comprehend the world as it is presented, and being (Cohen et al. 2000).

The hermeneutic circle is a way to critically analyze or explain an utterance, text, or action. It involves moving back and forth between the whole and the parts of an utterance, text, or action until the researcher understands or accounts for the meaning of strange passages and of the whole. In this process, the interpreter's self-understanding and sociohistorical location neither affects nor is affected by the effort to interpret meaning (Schwandt 2001).

Participatory action research

Participatory action research is a social process of collaborative learning. Together, researchers as well as community groups change the practices by which they interact in a world where, for better or worse, people live with the consequences of one another's actions (De Koning & Martin 1996; Kemmis & McTaggart 2005). This alternative philosophy of social research, often associated with social transformation in the Third World, has its roots in liberation theology and neo-Marxist approaches to community development and human rights activism (Kemmis & McTaggart 2005).

Action research began with an idea attributed to Kurt Lewin (1890–1947), who was born in Poland but later emigrated to the USA, who is considered to be the father of modern social psychology. His work in the 1940s found expression in the charitable Tavistock Institute of Human Relations. Founded in 1947, the institute sought 'ways to apply psychoanalytic and open systems concepts to group and organisational life' (Tavistock Institute). Lewin's earliest publications are about community action programs. He argued that social problems, rather than a scientist's own theoretical interest, should be the impulse for social research.

Other participatory action researchers have included the physician Jacob Moreno in Vienna, the American educator Stephen Corey, the British educators John Elliott and Clem Adelman, and Paulo Freire, Orlando Fals Borda, Rajesh Tandon, Anisur Rahman, and Marja-Liisa Swantz (Reason 1994; De Koning & Martin 1996; Schwandt 2001; Kemmis & McTaggart 2005).

Three attributes distinguish participatory action research from conventional research: shared ownership of research projects, community-based analysis of social problems, and an orientation toward community action (Kemmis & McTaggart 2005). Participatory action research is inquiry carried out by or with organization or community insiders, but never on them (Herr & Anderson 2005). Participation can be in the form of cooption, compliance, consultation, cooperation, colearning, or collective action (Cornwall 1996).

Researchers in the participatory action tradition study, reframe and reconstruct social practices (Kemmis & McTaggart 2005). The fruits of this learning process are changes in what people do, how they interact with the world and others, what people mean when they communicate, what they value, and discourses in which they understand and interpret their world. The process produces knowledge and action that are useful to a group. It aims to reach a voluntary consensus on what to do in a situation the group faces, empowers people at a deeper level by constructing and leveraging their knowledge, and encourages ongoing reflection and experimentation (Reason 1994; De Koning & Martin 1996; Schwandt 2001; Kemmis & McTaggart 2005).

Participatory action research is an alternative strategy for generating knowledge based on people's role in setting agendas, participating in data gathering and analysis, and controlling the use of outcomes (Reason 1994). It collects data through observation, interviews, action experiments, and cases and accounts written by participants (Schwandt 2001). The process is a spiral of self-reflective cycles: planning a change, taking action and observing the process and consequences of change, reflecting on these processes and consequences, replanning, acting and observing again, and reflecting again. These stages overlap, and initial plans quickly become obsolete in light of what is learned from experience. The idea is that changes occur either within the setting and/or within the researchers themselves (Schwandt 2001; Herr & Anderson 2005; Kemmis & McTaggart 2005).

Sampling and data saturation

Qualitative inquiry depends on purposefully selected samples. The researcher chooses individuals and contexts by asking: Who can give me the most and the best information about this topic? In which contexts will I be able to gather the most and best information (Mayan 2001)? In other words, respondents are selected based on their relevance to the research and their prior knowledge, not on their representativeness. The best participants are more receptive to an interview and more articulate. Morse (1994) describes a good participant as one who has the knowledge and experience the researcher needs, can reflect and articulate, has time to be interviewed, and is eager to participate.

Establishing explicit criteria for sample selection is critical (Morse & Field 1995; Schwandt 2001). Researchers may be helped in this task by first describing the study setting, who will be observed or interviewed, what the investigators intend to observe and what the interviews will focus on, and the evolving nature of events in the setting (Creswell 2003).

When should a researcher stop collecting data? When all of the data categories have been saturated. Saturation means no new or relevant data are emerging, the researcher has pursued all avenues or leads, and the story or theory is complete (Mayan 2001). A data category is dense and relationships between categories are well-established and validated (Strauss & Corbin 1990). Saturation has occurred when the researcher is very familiar with the setting or routine – perhaps even bored, feeling as if he or she has 'seen it all' (Morse 1994, p. 226).

Among the factors that determine how large a sample must be in order to reach saturation are the quality of data (are transcripts legible or audiotapes clear?), the study scope (broad versus narrow), whether the topic is clear and information can be easily obtained, the amount of useful information participants provide, the number of interviews per participant, whether shadowed data (participant reports on another's experience) are to be collected, and the study design and qualitative strategy (Morse 2000a; Mayan 2001).

Textual analyses

A text can consist of words or phrases or more lengthy segments (Schwandt 2001). There are four integral processes in textual analyses: comprehending, synthesizing, theorizing, and recontextualizing (Morse & Field 1995). These processes occur more or less sequentially. Thus, data analysis in qualitative inquiry is a systematic pattern of data collection–analysis–collection–analysis (Morse 1999) until saturation has been achieved. The researcher:

- Observes patterns in the data;
- Asks questions about those patterns;
- Forms conjectures;
- Confirms or refutes conjectures;

- Collects data from specific individuals on targeted topics;
- Continuously analyzes data;
- Asks additional questions;
- Seeks more data; and
- Does further analysis by sorting, questioning, thinking about, and constructing and testing conjectures (Morse 1999).

Circular analysis does not apply to data gathered from semi-structured or focus-group interviews. Rather, it takes place after all of the interviews are completed. Each question comprises a category of data, and the answers to questions are studied together (Morse 2000b; Mayan 2001).

There is a continuum of methods for analyzing textual data. On one end are methods (content analysis and objective hermeneutics) that emphasize content or what was said; on the other end are methods (conversation analysis and discourse analysis) that emphasize form or how something was said. Narrative analysis incorporates both content and form (Schwandt 2001). Thematic analysis (looking for themes), semantic analysis (language), and content analysis (e.g. categories, constructs, domains) have proliferated in recent years (Morse & Field 1995).

Content analysis, which applies to most qualitative inquiries, consists of coding the data, categorizing them into main and sub-categories, labeling the categories, integrating the categories into themes, and integrating all of the data (Mayan 2001). There are two types of content analysis: manifest and latent. In manifest content analysis, researchers look for specific words used or ideas expressed (Morse & Field 1995). In latent content analysis, they identify, code, and categorize primary patterns in the data (Patton 1990; Henning 2004). The investigators seek to understand the meaning of specific passages of text within the context of all the data (Mayan 2001).

Summary

In qualitative inquiries, researchers collect rich and in-depth data, interpret and synthesize the information, and gain a true understanding of a phenomenon. Strategies include grounded theory, historical, and case study research, and ethnography, phenomenology, hermeneutics, and participatory action, each of which is guided by the kinds of questions investigators seek to answer. All of the strategies rely on purposefully selected samples. Key considerations in sampling are explicit criteria for selecting study participants and knowing how many participants will be necessary to achieve saturation. Analyzing textual data entails a systematic pattern of data collection, analysis, more data collection, and more analysis. Qualitative inquiry not only sheds light on a phenomenon within a particular context, but also is a fulfilling and unforgettable experience for the investigator.

Note

1 'Strategy' is the preferred term in this discussion. Other authors use 'method,' 'methodology,' or 'approach' to mean generally the same thing.

References

Atkinson, P. & Hammersley, M. (1998) Ethnography and participant observation. In N.K. Denzin & Y.S. Lincoln (Eds) *Strategies of qualitative inquiry*. Thousand Oaks, CA: Sage Publications.

Bernard, H.R. (1988) *Research methods in cultural anthropology*. Newbury Park, CA: Sage Publications.

Bernard, H.R. (2000) *Social research methods: Qualitative and quantitative approaches*. Thousand Oaks, CA: Sage Publications.

Bogdan, R.C. & Biklen, S.K. (1992) *Qualitative research for education: An introduction to theory and methods*. Needham Heights, MA: Allyn & Bacon.

Charmaz, K. (2005) Grounded theory in the 21st century: Applications for advancing social justice studies. In N.K. Denzin & Y.S. Lincoln (Eds) *The Sage handbook of qualitative research*, 3rd Edn. Thousand Oaks, CA: Sage Publications.

Cohen, M.Z., Kahn, D.L. & Steeve, R.H. (2000) *Hermeneutic phenomenological research*. Thousand Oaks, CA: Sage Publications.

Cornwall, A. (1996) Towards participatory practice: Participatory rural appraisal (PRA) and the participatory process. In K. De Koning & M. Martin (Eds) *Participatory research in health: Issues and experiences*. London: Zed Books.

Creswell, J.W. (1998) *Qualitative inquiry and research design: Choosing among five traditions*. Thousand Oaks, CA: Sage Publications.

Creswell, J.W. (2003) *Research design: Qualitative, quantitative, and mixed methods approaches*, 2nd Edn. Thousand Oaks, CA: Sage Publications.

De Koning, K. & Martin, M. (1996) *Participatory research in health: Issues and experiences*. London: Zed Books.

Denzin, N.K. & Lincoln, Y.S. (Eds) (2005) *The Sage handbook of qualitative research*, 3rd Edn. Thousand Oaks, CA: Sage Publications.

De Vos, A.S., Strydom, H., Fouche, C.B. & Delport, C.S.L. (2005) *Research at grass roots for the social sciences and human service professions*, 3rd Edn. Pretoria: Van Schaik Publishers.

Glaser, B.G. & Strauss, A.L. (1967) *The discovery of grounded theory: Strategies for qualitative research*. Chicago: Aldine Publishing.

Henning, E. (2004) *Finding your way in qualitative research*. Pretoria: Van Schaik Publishers.

Herr, K. & Anderson, G.L. (2005) *The action research dissertation: A guide for students and faculty*. Thousand Oaks, CA: Sage Publications.

Kemmis, S. & McTaggart, R. (2005) Participatory action research: Communicative action and the public sphere. In N.K. Denzin & Y.S. Lincoln (Eds) *The Sage handbook of qualitative research*, 3rd Edn. Thousand Oaks, CA: Sage Publications.

Mark, R. (1996) *Research made simple: A handbook for social workers*. London: Sage Publications.

Mayan, M.J. (2001) *An introduction to qualitative methods: A training module for students and professionals*. Edmonton: International Institute for Qualitative Methodology, University of Alberta.

Morse, J.M. (1994) Designing funded qualitative research. In N.K. Denzin & Y.S. Lincoln (Eds) *Handbook of qualitative research*. Thousand Oaks, CA: Sage Publications.

Morse, J.M. (1999) Myth 19: Qualitative inquiry is not systematic. *Qualitative Health Research* **9**(5), 573.

Morse, J.M. (2000a) Determining sample size. *Qualitative Health Research* **10**(1), 3.

Morse, J.M. (2000b) *Principles of qualitative inquiry*. Nursing 560 (course). Edmonton: University of Alberta.

Morse, J.M. & Field, P.A. (1995) *Qualitative research methods for health professionals*, 2nd Edn. Thousand Oaks, CA: Sage Publications.

Patton, M.Q. (1990) *Qualitative evaluation and research methods*, 2nd Edn. Thousand Oaks, CA: Sage Publications.

Potter, W.J. (1996) *An analysis of thinking and research about qualitative methods.* Mahwah, NJ: Lawrence Erlbaum Associates.

Reason, P. (1994) Three approaches to participatory inquiry. In N.K. Denzin & Y.S. Lincoln (Eds) *Handbook of qualitative research.* Thousand Oaks, CA: Sage Publications.

Roper, J.M. & Shapira, J. (2000) *Ethnography in nursing research.* Thousand Oaks, CA: Sage Publications.

Schwandt, T.A. (2001) *Dictionary of qualitative inquiry*, 2nd Edn. Thousand Oaks, CA: Sage Publications.

Stake, R.E. (1995) *The art of case study research.* Thousand Oaks, CA: Sage Publications.

Stake, R.E. (2005) Qualitative case studies. In N.K. Denzin & Y.S. Lincoln (Eds) *The Sage handbook of qualitative research*, 3rd Edn. Thousand Oaks, CA: Sage Publications.

Strauss, A. & Corbin, J. (1990) *Basics of qualitative research: Grounded theory procedures and techniques.* Newbury Park, CA: Sage Publications.

Strauss, A. & Corbin, J. (1994) Grounded theory methodology. In N.K. Denzin & Y.S. Lincoln (Eds) *Handbook of qualitative research.* Thousand Oaks, CA: Sage Publications.

Tavistock Institute. Our history. www.tavinstitute.org/about/our_history.php.

Tedlock, B. (2005) The observation of participation and the emergence of public ethnography. In N.K. Denzin & Y.S. Lincoln (Eds) *The Sage handbook of qualitative research*, 3rd Edn. Thousand Oaks, CA: Sage Publications.

Tuchman, G. (1994) Historical social science. In N.K. Denzin & Y.S. Lincoln (Eds) *Handbook of qualitative research.* Thousand Oaks, CA: Sage Publications.

Van Manen, M. (1997) *Researching lived experience: Human science for an action sensitive pedagogy*, 2nd Edn. Toronto: Althouse Press.

Wolcott, H.T. (1999) *Ethnography: A way of seeing.* Walnut Creek, CA: AltaMira Press.

Chapter 15
Interpretive data management and analysis

Roberta S. Rehm

Introduction

One of the defining, fundamental assumptions of nursing is that health is the result of multiple internal and external influences – genetic, physiologic, social, spiritual, and environmental – and that nurses' mission is to interact with human beings and communities in a holistic manner that acknowledges and respects these influences (Flaskerud & Halloran 1980; Potter & Frisch 2007). Interpretive researchers illuminate such influences and examine in-depth the contexts surrounding particular social and cultural situations (Willis 2007). Nurse researchers seek to facilitate systematic understanding of the nature of human behavior and experience in relation to health, sickness, crisis, and life circumstances (Hagadorn & Zahourek 2007).

Although the term 'interpretive' is sometimes used interchangeably with 'qualitative,' not all qualitative research is interpretive (Sandelowski 2000). Some qualitative investigators interpret their findings and put them in context, while others literally and strictly describe them. Most interpretive researchers accept that reality is never completely discoverable and that participants and investigators socially construct reality during research (constructivism). Instead of searching for irrefutable truths, interpretive researchers seek to understand experiences, situations, and social relationships (Power 2004; Willis 2007).

Underlying paradigms

A research paradigm is a generally accepted set of assumptions in a profession or scholarly community that captures foundational beliefs and practices. For the most part, adherents agree on the nature of truth or reality, the possibility of objectivity, and the nature of evidence. Although there is some controversy about which and how many paradigms in nursing research are firmly established, most scholars recognize several types, including post-positivist, interpretive, and critical paradigms (Weaver & Olson, 2006).

Post-positivist

Post-positivism developed as philosophers realized that increasing scientific knowledge made the search for absolute truths untenable. Earlier, logical positivists had sought answers to scientific questions that were value-free and perfectly objective. Post-positivists accept that objectivity is desirable but never perfect, and that truth can be approximated but not necessarily verified. Truth and reality, they acknowledge, are complicated and knowable only imperfectly; therefore, claims about reality must be modest and subjected to critical examination.

Post-positivists seek objective knowledge and evidence of repetitive and predictable patterns that govern or influence the physical and social worlds. They may use these regularities of nature and human social life to explain causation or association, and to predict and explain observable phenomena. Truth, they believe, is independent of the observer and researchers should strive to be objective. Controlling investigator bias and structuring studies to eliminate extraneous variables that could influence findings is an important part of assuring rigorous research (Weaver & Olson 2006).

Quantitative, post-positivist studies are often designed to build and test theory.[1] Adherents believe that accurate theories could explain both observable phenomena and those that are not yet observable (for example, because of technologic limitations). A sound theory, by this reasoning, could predict reality. Adherents assume that metaphysical phenomena are outside the scientific realm.

The post-positivist approach requires precision, logic, and evidence in order to be able to draw firm conclusions, which are usually derived deductively. Scientists studying health and patient care in this paradigm view randomized clinical trials, with control and experimental groups, as the highest form of research. Data, which are often quantitative, come from measurable phenomena. However, researchers' perceptions are not considered to be wholly detached from the inquiry, and many investigators accept inferential data, such as self-reports, as legitimate. Post-positivists, unlike interpretive researchers, often try to standardize data collection tools and conditions, as well as analysis methods, to maximize objectivity, minimize the possibility of bias, and increase their ability to generalize findings (Letourneau & Allen 1999).

Interpretive

In contrast to post-positivists, interpretive researchers assume that reality is dynamic, there are multiple truths, and truth is relative, depending on the particular situation; truth even differs among individuals or groups in similar circumstances (Becker 2001). This is a post-modern way of thinking. Indeed, post-modern movements among scholars in a wide variety of disciplines have influenced the assumptions underlying interpretive research (Cheek 2000). Interpretive scientists do not assume that truth and reality are ever completely knowable. Rather, they believe that truth resides within individuals and is shaped by ongoing social and group dynamics that change as circumstances evolve.

Interpretive research is inductive: conclusions and findings are based on analysis of data, which can come from a variety of sources, including interviews, observations, documents, or artifacts (Holloway & Wheeler 2002). Investigators collect data in real-life situations, not in the laboratory or a controlled environment (Murphy 2005). The context of human behavior and social situations is complex, so instead of trying to control the influences and variations that might cause differences in experience or perception, interpretive researchers explore them.

Interpretive researchers are commonly influenced by constructivism, symbolic interaction, or other German and American philosophical traditions whose research goal is to gain a deep understanding of everyday life experiences in context. These underpinnings lead to the belief that reality, arising from interactions between individuals and groups, is socially constructed, rather than absolute or subjective, and should be interpreted self-reflectively (Bailey & Tilley 2002; Clarke 2005). In their view, understanding the meaning that particular situations have for study participants is important because participants' actions, behaviors, and decisions arise from the meaning they attach to things, persons, or situations (Becker 2001). Investigators acknowledge their own influence on the research process and do not think total objectivity is possible (Hegelund 2005). They examine all sources of influence and, through reflective thought and writing in the analysis, assess their personal impact on the study. This contrasts sharply with quantitative methods, which seek generalizable rules or patterns – often in tightly controlled circumstances – that can lead to predictable and controllable outcomes.

Practical use of knowledge derived from interpretive research is growing. According to Sandelowski (2004), uses include the development of culturally appropriate research tools and interventions that are tailored to specific situations and that are feasible and acceptable to patients. Interpretive research also provides direction for clinical evaluation projects and further studies.

Theory sometimes informs the work of interpretive investigators, providing foundational concepts or serving as a starting point to investigate particular topics that are central to a theory. Interpretive research may contribute to the development of theory – not only through grounded theory research, the explicit goal of which is theorizing, but also through the development and application of concepts that help explain or illustrate the context of findings in other methodologies, such as ethnography or phenomenology. Links between clinical situations and theory can be fostered through interpretive field research that encourages conceptual thinking, furthers theoretical discussion of clinical experiences, and posits conceptual links between practice experiences and research findings (Schwartz-Barcott et al. 2002).

Critical

Some interpretive researchers favor the critical paradigm, which is rooted in Marxism (Willis 2007). Truth and reality, they believe, are shaped by social, political, cultural, gender, sexual, and economic factors. Scholars with a critical perspective are explicitly ideological and political, and view such factors as often oppressive (Weaver & Olson 2006). They seek to remove oppressive influences and empower oppressed people.

Although other interpretive researchers generally respect critical methodologies, they usually are not explicitly ideological and political. Instead, their goal is to improve understanding of the complexities and ambiguities of human experience.

Interpretive methods and procedures

A variety of qualitative research methodologies – such as phenomenology, ethnography, symbolic interaction, and grounded theory – rely on an interpretive paradigm (Slaughter et al. 2007; Willis 2007). Other methodologies include historical, feminist, and narrative research, and discourse analysis. Whether a study is interpretive or descriptive depends on the assumptions of the investigators, the design of data collection and analysis, and the study's goals and the products it disseminates (Sandelowski 2000).

Methodologies vary in terms of whether they are more interpretive or more descriptive. (Holloway & Todres 2003). In phenomenology, for example, two of the best known variations are Heidegerrian phenomenology (interpretive) and Husserlian phenomenology (descriptive). Anthropologic and sociologic ethnography and grounded theory have become more interpretive over time as investigators adopted post-modern and constructivist perspectives (Charmaz 2006). Methodologies evolve over time as scholars challenge, extend, and push the work of their predecessors in new directions (Wolf 1992; Fine 1995; Clarke 2005).

There are no overarching procedures or guidelines that interpretive researchers universally follow (Silverman 2006). Each interpretive method has its own tradition. However, the different methods do have some things in common.

All researchers first identify a problem – perhaps something they noticed in clinical practice or read about in a previous study – that warrants investigation. Then they review the literature to learn what has been published about their topic of interest, identify gaps in knowledge, and ensure that the time, effort, and expense of a new study will be justified.

Although some qualitative researchers claim they skip literature reviews to avoid 'contaminating' their initial openness and objectivity, most do thorough reviews. Complete objectivity, interpretive researchers know, is not possible.

In addition, all researchers must leap the same pragmatic hurdles. For example, they must obtain funding and undergo an ethical review of their study proposal.

Proposals

Investigators should develop formal proposals that reflect careful thought and planning because influential people, including potential collaborators, reviewers for funding agencies, and members of ethical review boards, must be able to clearly understand a prospective project (Knafl & Deatrick 2005; Ungar 2006).

A good purpose statement and specific aims or research questions convey the idea that the researchers will foster understanding of particular social situations or processes, analyze meanings that drive actions or decisions, and produce an in-depth, or 'thick,' description (Geertz 1987; Beitz & Bliss 2005; Ayers 2007).

One of the strengths of qualitative research is the ability to respond to emerging data and tentative findings as the study proceeds, so interpretive researchers must be flexible enough to refocus their aims or questions during data collection. However, they also must present sufficient details at the outset to convince others that the study is important, even necessary.

The background and significance section in the proposal cites the known contextual factors that influence the study situation and/or population. It usually makes the case that the topic is important because it causes suffering; requires large expenditures of time, money, or other resources; or the results could lead to better health or higher quality of life.

The proposal then specifically describes the procedures for sampling, data collection and analysis, rigorous control of the research, and ethical considerations (Vivar et al. 2007). Often, proposals also contain sections citing the researchers' qualifications, any preliminary findings on the topic from earlier studies, and the budget.

Sampling

Because interpretive researchers are especially interested in contextual factors that influence daily life and social situations, they usually seek participants who have first-hand knowledge of and experience with the circumstances to be studied. This is called purposive or purposeful sampling (Coyne 1997). It may narrowly focus on only one type of participant if the purpose is to gain an in-depth understanding of a situation from one perspective, as in phenomenologic studies. Or it may include several participant types, each with a unique perspective, as in ethnographic or sociologic field studies.

Another approach is theoretical sampling, which grounded theorists employ. Investigators select participants who have very specific experiences or knowledge that will contribute to a theory under development, or participants who can provide feedback on preliminary concepts the researchers have constructed (Higginbottom 2004; Corbin & Strauss 2007).

Interpretive researchers generally halt sampling and data collection when they conclude that two conditions have been met: the interpretation is well developed and new data would likely be redundant. This method of determining sample size, called saturation, must be explained in the proposal. Researchers typically estimate the sample size – often by providing a range, such as 15–20 participants – based on when they expect saturation will be reached. The literature suggests that many qualitative projects reach saturation with 12–25 participants, but final sample sizes vary depending on the number of interviews or observations, and on a study's particular purposes (Tucket 2004).

Recruitment

Before data collection begins, researchers must plan how they will recruit participants, a step that involves ethical considerations. Although subjects in interpretive studies rarely face physical risks, researchers must guard the privacy, autonomy, and emotional well-being of prospective participants and those they select (Davies & Dodd 2002; Hewitt 2007).

One effective recruitment strategy that nurse researchers often use is collaboration with clinical partners who are also interested in the study topic.

Clinicians make the initial contact by telling patients about a research project and the need for willing subjects. Researchers then approach interested patients to provide more details and obtain informed consent if patients agree to participate. This strategy protects the privacy of prospective participants because researchers initially have little or no specific information about them. Ethically, all participants must be assured that their contribution is completely voluntary and worth their time and effort (Hewitt 2007).

Interviews

Interviews, observations, and reviews of materials such as documents or cultural artifacts are typical data sources in interpretive studies (Holloway & Wheeler 2002; Miller & Alvarado 2005). Among these sources, the most common and important one is interviews (DiCicco-Bloom & Crabtree 2006).

Researchers usually prepare a preliminary set of questions, called an interview guide, to elicit information from participants. In semi-structured interviews, they typically begin with open-ended questions that invite broad responses, then pose more focused questions to follow up on respondents' answers and probe the topic more deeply (Dearnley 2005). Surveys and questionnaires, in contrast, often pose close-ended or forced-choice questions that require a definitive response, such as 'yes' or 'no,' or selection of an answer on a scale of perhaps 1–5 reflecting strong agreement or strong disagreement with a statement.

Interpretive researchers glean textual information rather than numerical data from interviews, looking for similarities and variations within certain contexts. They seek participants' perspectives and are not concerned with quantifying answers or ensuring statistical significance. Individual interviews often vary, as questions may evoke unique responses, which in turn prompt researchers to ask questions tailored to the interviewee. Good interviewers express empathy through verbal and body language, and contemplate the concerns and priorities reflected in interviewees' answers. An ability to respond to participants' concerns is much more important than rigid adherence to the interview guide or creating similar conditions for all informants (Willis 2007).

Many interviewer-, participant-, and context-related factors affect interview quality (Birks et al. 2007). One is the interviewer's communication skills, especially the ability to establish trust and rapport. Nurse researchers often ask participants about very private or personal matters, such as living with illness, loss, or grief. Regardless of whether the process evokes short-term sadness, anger, or other distress, informants should have a positive experience. For example, in a study about palliative care needs, Hynson et al. (2006) asked bereaved parents what it was like to discuss their child and the grief they felt within 2 years of the child's death. Parents were very positive about participating in the study, even if they found the interview to be upsetting. They cited the compassion of the interviewer; the sensitive invitation to participate; their sense of control over the time, place, and pace of the interview; and how, in telling their story to a sympathetic listener, other families experiencing a similar loss might benefit. In such situations, some interviewers are prepared to offer referrals for follow-up support if participants feel they need it.

Other important interviewing skills are truly listening to what participants say, sensing when it is appropriate to ask another question or wait, and allowing silences while informants gather their thoughts or work through their emotions. Adept interviewers also probe for clarification or further development of participants' narratives or analysis of their own situation (Dearnley 2005). Although nurse researchers frequently have expert clinical knowledge about a topic, they must keep in mind that the purpose of interviews is not clinical care, but rather understanding participants' lives and context of experience (Hewitt 2007). Interviewers do not have to pretend they are naïve or avoid speaking with participants about other topics. But they must be able to keep the general focus on the subject matter and participants' narratives, and know how to maintain the flow of discussion.

Participants' level of anxiety, language proficiency, and desire to please the interviewer may affect interview quality. Birks et al. (2007) note that these factors can be particularly important in cross-cultural research or in interviews with people from cultures other than the researcher's. Because interviews take place in the field, the setting and conditions will likely vary. Interruptions and distractions are common, but they may produce additional data.

Developing interview skills requires considerable, intense practice. One helpful learning strategy is to study interview transcripts with skilled mentors to identify opportunities other investigators missed for a follow-up question, and to identify ways to put participants at ease, such as offering verbal or non-verbal encouragement.

Observation

Formal or informal observation is part of most interpretive studies (Angrosino & Mays de Perez 2000). Interpretive researchers are keenly aware of their surroundings as they gather data. They typically record their observations in field notes, journals, or other written forms so they can later retrieve the information, incorporate it into other data, and analyze everything (Wolfinger 2002).

A study's goals and methodology, and perhaps circumstances in the field, determine the degree to which observers immerse themselves in the study environment. Some researchers simply observe and record what is happening around them, as in interviews and focus groups. Others actively partake in the setting, which enables them to closely observe daily occurrences (Emerson & Pollner 2001).

Observation may be the primary data collection method, or observations may supplement other data to create a fuller or more nuanced understanding (Angrosino & Mays de Perez 2000). Observation may be particularly helpful in gathering data about participants who cannot be interviewed – for example, very young children, or people who are not verbal. In the past, cultural anthropologists resided in far-away locations to learn about the beliefs, traits, and habits of isolated, unfamiliar populations whose culture seemed quite exotic. Anthropologist Margaret Mead (2001) became famous when she lived among islanders in the early 20th century and described adolescent behavior in *Coming of Age in Samoa*. She claimed to have adopted the islanders' habits and to have won their trust and confidence by joining them in numerous activities, which enabled her to write a definitive and factual account of cultural phenomena. Participants have disputed Mead's and other definitive cultural accounts, saying they shared only partial information or even deceived researchers at times (Wolf 1992).

Over the years, complete immersion in the research setting fell out of favor as field workers realized that knowledge gained in this manner is only one type of information – that it is based on certain circumstances and the relationship between researchers and informants, and that the information by no means reflects definitive truth. Today, field workers take a more nuanced approach. They recognize that their work will result only in a partial depiction of circumstances in a particular time and place. Furthermore, gaining access to information from interviews, observation, shared activities, or casual conversation is a matter of negotiation with participants, and a product of the level of trust and respect between them and researchers (Borbasi et al. 2005).

Observation enables researchers to gain a deeper understanding of a social situation and to broaden their knowledge of contextual factors that have a role in different situations (Willis 2007). Observers describe both physical settings and human behavior, including human interactions. Structures, artwork, provisions for comfort, privacy protections, or other things that facilitate or inhibit activities are all settings. Equally important may be the absence of things, such as toys in a home with children; people; or events that a researcher might expect would occur under certain circumstances.

Researchers may focus on people's daily activities or on the people themselves, by means of interviews or observation. Observing people during interviews – for example, the clothing they wear and their body language, eye contact, bearing, and style of communication with the investigator, family members, and others – provides clues about their comfort in a setting, their self-identity, or their ability to interact. Regardless of whether observation is the only approach or one of multiple approaches, it adds depth to words and explanations, and yields a better understanding of participants' daily lives (Emerson & Pollner 2001).

Foremost among ethical considerations is that observation should be open (Angrosino & Mays de Perez 2000; Emerson & Pollner 2001). Even if observers are fully participating in the activities around them, they should not attempt to hide their purpose and may feel obliged to remind people of it. Observation is open and honest when investigators take notes in plain view, ask questions as activities unfold, and discuss the research with newcomers.

Data analysis

Data analysis is the heart of qualitative research. Interpretive researchers gain a deep understanding of their subject by deliberately, systematically, and thoroughly reviewing data (Silverman 2006). Common products of interpretive data analysis are 'thick description' (Geertz 1987) or theory grounded in data (Glaser & Strauss 1967). In-depth descriptions and theories may include analyses of social processes in daily life – processes that often create or reflect meanings that underpin the decisions or actions of study participants (Benner et al. 1996; Becker 2001; Clarke, 2005).

Reflexivity and iterative processing are important, linked concepts in interpretive analysis. In the post-modern tradition, reflexivity is acknowledgment of one's own biases, desires, and expectations in research (Denzin 2000; Mauthner & Doucet 2003). Iterative processing means research unfolds in repetitive waves of data collection and analysis (Crist & Tanner 2003; Charmaz 2006).

Interpretive researchers do not believe in absolute objectivity nor seek it when they collect and analyze data. Instead, they try to understand their contributions to and effects on the conduct of research (Emerson & Pollner 2001; Borbasi et al. 2005). They accomplish this through self-reflection, or reflexivity. In field notes or memos, they reflect on their own backgrounds, experiences, and responses to the current participants or situations the investigators are encountering (Wolfinger 2002). By doing so, they become aware of biases or other factors that may limit what they hear from participants or that prevent them from investigating contextual influences on the study topic.

In iterative processing, analysis begins soon after data collection begins. Investigators continuously assess what they are finding and the data-gathering method. Iterative processing enables them to respond to priorities or topics that arise in the course of research and to revise interview questions or observation guides as necessary. They may decide to add other data collection methods if early results are interesting enough to warrant further investigation.

Reflexivity and iterative processing encourage ethical practices. They can expose self-centered or coercive motives for design decisions, and give investigators an opportunity to alter or correct the research process if necessary (Borbasi et al. 2005; Hewitt 2007).

Analytical procedures vary among interpretive research methodologies, and also vary among investigators who apply the same methodology. Interpretive analysts use multiple analysis techniques, but they cannot presume that any particular one is the best or the only effective way to achieve rigor (Coffey & Atkinson 1996). The most important thing is that the analysis systematically incorporates all significant variations in the data and fully considers the contextual influences (Silverman 2006).

There are several common elements in qualitative analysis. Grounded theory researchers and ethnographers prioritize and select data that will undergo further analysis. They usually do this by assigning codes to segments of data, breaking down the data and classifying them in conceptual categories for focused analysis, and linking the main concepts into a coherent or understandable whole (Coffey & Atkinson 1996; Silverman 2006; Corbin & Strauss 2007). Other interpretive traditions, such as phenomenology, prefer not to break down data, but rather keep the information intact so researchers can gain a holistic and contextual understanding (Benner et al. 1996; Crist & Tanner 2003).

Nearly all analytical techniques have their own unique vocabulary. However, common features are repetitive reading of data, recursive consideration of the meaning of words or participants' actions, comparison of a participant's data with the aggregate data, and development of an overall narrative.

Software

Among the computer programs that nurse researchers most often use to facilitate qualitative data analysis are ATLAS.ti and NVivo. These products make it much easier to manage large data sets or complex research projects with multiple parts, mostly by enabling retrieval of particular data segments, which are usually conceptual units such as words, several lines of dialogue, or a participant's story. The software enables segments to be linked to researchers' written analyses (Wickham & Woods 2005). Teams can share individual members' analyses, then merge the analyses or work cooperatively through each iteration. While ATLAS.ti and NVivo can be difficult to learn and cumbersome to use (Weitzman 1999), their popularity is growing.

Procedures

Analysis often begins by reading a data segment and trying to get a sense of what is happening within it (Coffey & Atkinson 1996; Crist & Tanner 2003). The size of segments varies. Many grounded theorists assign codes to very short segments, such as a word or line of text, while phenomenologists use codes to mark larger segments, such as a story about an event. Many interpretive researchers first read the entire transcript of an interview to grasp the big picture, then write a short summary. The summary condenses a participant's story into an easily read narrative identifying salient historical and current events, priorities, and concerns. Summaries can later serve as reminders of important information in the transcript and allow a quick comparison of participants' experiences as analysis proceeds.

Coding, either manually or with the help of software, enables researchers to organize, manage, and retrieve data, which may be quite extensive. In open coding, investigators place a distinctive shorthand next to an idea or event in the transcript. This may include 'in vivo' codes – words inserted in the transcript to summarize text. Grounded theorists often code each word or line in documents as a way to understand fine gradations of meaning. Others assign codes to larger chunks of data, such as those related to concepts or ideas. Codes can be highly conceptual, identifying and linking important concepts or ideas in a transcript, or merely mechanical to allow retrieval of data at a later time. The advent of computer-assisted analysis has encouraged even holistically oriented researchers to develop a coding system for retrieving and manipulating smaller data segments (Wickham & Woods 2005).

In later stages of analysis, qualitative researchers often combine the open codes they initially assigned into categories representing experiences or concepts across the population of participants. This enables them to compare early bits of data with data they subsequently collect from the same and other participants, a process that grounded theorists call constant comparative analysis. Grounded theorists sometimes use higher levels of coding than other interpretive researchers. Axial coding, for example, specifies the properties and dimensions of a category and relates categories to sub-categories. Theoretical coding helps a theory evolve by noting possible relationships between data categories developed earlier in the process (Charmaz 2006).

During data analysis, qualitative researchers hone their thinking and share their thoughts with other members of the team by writing memos (Montgomery & Bailey 2007). Memos can be informal, minimally structured notes in which the analyst explores or defines an idea in more detail, or they can be more organized presentations arguing for a particular interpretation of the data or a tentative conclusion. Recording analytical thoughts and ideas often helps investigators connect concepts and think more deeply about the story or circumstance under discussion, resulting in links between participants or common themes in the aggregate data (Van Manen 2006). Analytical teams sometimes write memos to clarify strategies and explain processes to each other. Memos also can organize the long and multifaceted evolution and construction of the final interpretation of results. Many computer programs contain memo-writing tools that help prepare notes about chunks of data or link particular codes or data categories (Wickham & Woods 2005).

Interpretive researchers realize that their findings are just one version or representation of reality in a particular context. They must carefully consider which voices dominate, which data to include, and how to portray the context (Sandelowski 1998). Because inaccurate, slanted, or incomplete findings may influence policy-makers' or clinicians' decisions regarding funding or health care interventions, ethical researchers try to ensure that their results are placed in context and fully explained.

The final data analysis furthers the understanding of a study topic and its context, and assesses factors that affect both the similarities and differences among participants. It often includes a reflexive statement acknowledging and describing influences the researchers knowingly or possibly brought to bear on the study (Mauthner & Doucet 2003). For example, nurses frequently have clinical experiences that may influence their interactions with study participants.

Rigor and integrity

Interpretive research enhances rigor, or the quality and strength of the findings and the methods used to achieve them, and integrity by being systematic and by incorporating design, data-collection, and analysis procedures that ensure fair and comprehensive consideration of the data. Integrity means the study design respects the experience and voices of participants, the researchers acknowledge the impact they may have had on the findings, and the results resonate with everyday life and may be useful to others.

By way of asserting rigor, early qualitative scholars used terminology and principles analogous to those in quantitative research. Lincoln and Guba (1985) defined the qualitative concepts 'credibility,' 'dependability,' 'confirmability,' and 'transferability' in terms that respectively mirror the quantitative concepts 'internal validity,' 'reliability,' 'objectivity,' and 'generalizability.'

More recently, however, interpretive researchers have asserted that because truth and reality are multiple and relative, rigor should demonstrate thorough, thoughtful, and meaningful collection and analysis of data (Angen 2000). Preoccupation with procedures to ensure rigor, some qualitative scholars have cautioned, could interfere with the creativity and flexibility that are hallmarks of interpretive studies (Sandelowski 1993). Researchers have designed several alternative schemas for assessing the rigor of qualitative studies. These schemas encourage investigators to pay attention to procedures and processes, thereby ensuring systematic and ethical studies and believable findings (Angen 2000; Whittemore et al. 2001; Davies & Dodd 2002).

There are no universally accepted criteria for rigor, although researchers commonly use several procedures to enhance it. Most investigators collect significant quantities of data and stop only when they have reached saturation. In addition, qualitative researchers often use more than one data source, such as multiple settings or categories of informants – a technique called triangulation (Willis 2007). Methodologic triangulation involves multiple data collection methods, such as interviews, observations, and focus groups. Investigator triangulation occurs when members of a research team collaborate and share important aspects of data analysis and interpretation. In theoretical triangulation, investigators explain findings in alternative ways and compare the different interpretations, seeking the best fit for the data they gathered. They often solicit input from participants by way of comparing participants' intent and analysis with researchers' interpretations. In this process, investigators must understand that multiple versions of truth may coexist and that no single version is correct. They may also ask peers or other experts in the field to review the findings and assess them for believability, coherence, and resonance (Whittemore et al. 2001).

Conclusions

Interpretive research is a distinct form of qualitative investigation based on a post-modern perspective. Although there are different qualitative research methodologies, adherents agree that reality is situated, socially constructed, and dynamic; truth is never completely knowable; and the goal is to gain a deeper understanding of everyday life in context. To that end, investigators often collect data by reviewing other documents and materials, and by interviewing and/or observing people.

Interpretive researchers analyze data in a variety of ways, depending on the study's methodology. Analysis frequently includes management of data sets using a qualitative software program, coding of data, writing memos to communicate analyses, repeatedly assessing data, and comparing data from individual participants with aggregate data. Procedures such as reflexivity, methodologic and investigator triangulation, and discussing preliminary data interpretations with study participants help ensure the rigor and integrity of results.

Note

1 Qualitative research, in contrast, often does not seek to test a theory. Rather, it may try to build theory inductively.

References

Angen, M.J. (2000) Evaluating interpretive inquiry: Reviewing the validity debate and opening the dialogue. *Qualitative Health Research* **10**(3), 378–395.

Angrosino, M.V. & Mays de Perez, K.A. (2000) Rethinking observation: From method to context. In N.K. Denzin & Y.S. Lincoln (Eds) *Handbook of qualitative research* (pp. 673–702). Thousand Oaks, CA: Sage Publications.

Ayers, L. (2007) Qualitative research proposals. Part 1: Posing the problem. *Journal of Wound, Ostomy and Continence Nursing* **34**(1), 30–32.

Bailey, P.H. & Tilley, S. (2002) Storytelling and the interpretation of meaning in qualitative research. *Journal of Advanced Nursing* **38**(6), 574–583.

Becker, H.S. (2001) The epistemology of qualitative research. In R.M. Emerson (Ed) *Contemporary fieldwork*, 2nd Edn (pp. 317–330). Prospect Heights, IL: Waveland Press.

Beitz, J.M. & Bliss, D.Z. (2005) Spotlight on research. Preparing a successful grant proposal. Part 1: Developing research aims and the significance of the project. *Journal of Wound, Ostomy and Continence Nursing* **32**(1), 16–18.

Benner, P., Tanner, C. & Chesla, C. (1996) Background and method. In P. Benner, C. Tanner & C. Chesla (Eds) *Expertise in nursing practice: Caring, clinical judgment and ethics* (pp. 351–372). New York: Springer.

Birks, M.J., Chapman, Y. & Francis, K. (2007) Breaching the wall: Interviewing people from other cultures. *Journal of Transcultural Nursing* **18**(2), 150–156.

Borbasi, S., Jackson, D. & Wilkes, L. (2005) Fieldwork in nursing research: Positionality, practicalities, and predicaments. *Journal of Advanced Nursing* **51**(5), 493–501.

Charmaz, K.C. (2006) *Constructing grounded theory: A practical guide through qualitative analysis.* Thousand Oaks, CA: Sage Publications.

Cheek, J. (2000) *Postmodern and poststructural approaches to nursing research.* Thousand Oaks, CA: Sage Publications.

Clarke, A. (2005) *Situational analysis: Grounded theory after the postmodern turn.* Thousand Oaks, CA: Sage Publications.

Coffey, A. & Atkinson, P. (1996) *Making sense of qualitative data: Complementary research strategies.* Thousand Oaks, CA: Sage Publications.

Corbin, J.M. & Strauss, A.L. (2007) *Basics of qualitative research: Techniques and procedures for developing grounded theory*, 3rd Edn. Thousand Oaks, CA: Sage Publications.

Coyne, I.T. (1997) Sampling in qualitative research. Purposeful and theoretical sampling: merging or clear boundaries? *Journal of Advanced Nursing* **26**(3), 623–630.

Crist, J.D. & Tanner, C.A. (2003) Interpretation/analysis methods in hermeneutic interpretive phenomenology. *Nursing Research* **52**(3), 202–205.

Davies, D. & Dodd, J. (2002) Qualitative research and the question of rigor. *Qualitative Health Research* **12**(2), 279–289.

Dearnley, C. (2005) A reflection on the use of semi-structured interviews. *Nurse Researcher* **13**(1), 19–28.

Denzin, N.K. (2000) The practices and politics of interpretation. In N.K. Denzin & Y.S. Lincoln (Eds) *Handbook of qualitative research* (pp. 897–922). Thousand Oaks, CA: Sage Publications.

DiCicco-Bloom, B. & Crabtree, B.F. (2006) The qualitative research interview. *Medical Education* **40**(4), 314–321.

Emerson, R.M. & Pollner, M. (2001) Constructing participant/observation relations. In R.M. Emerson (Ed) *Contemporary fieldwork*, 2nd Edn (pp. 239–259). Prospect Heights, IL: Waveland Press.

Fine, G.A. (1995) *A second Chicago school? The development of a postwar American sociology.* Chicago: University of Chicago Press.

Flaskerud, J.H. & Halloran, E.J. (1980) Areas of agreement in nursing theory development. *Advances in Nursing Science* **3**(1), 1–7.

Geertz, C. (1987) Deep play: Notes on the Balinese cockfight. In P. Rabinow & W.S. Sullivan (Eds) *Interpretive social science: A second look* (pp. 195–240). Berkeley: University of California Press.

Glaser, B.G. & Strauss, A.L. (1967) *The discovery of grounded theory: Strategies for qualitative research.* Chicago: Aldine.

Hagedorn, M.E. & Zahourek, R.P. (2007) Research paradigms and methods for investigating holistic nursing concerns. *Nursing Clinics of North America* **42**(2), 335–353.

Hegelund, A. (2005) Objectivity and subjectivity in the ethnographic method. *Qualitative Health Research* **15**(5), 647–668.

Hewitt, J. (2007) Ethical components of researcher–researched relationships in qualitative interviewing. *Qualitative Health Research* **17**(8), 1149–1159.

Higginbottom, G.M.A. (2004) Sampling issues in qualitative research. *Nurse Researcher* **12**(1), 7–19.

Holloway, I. & Todres, L. (2003) The status of method: Flexibility, consistency and coherence. *Qualitative Research* **3**(3), 345–357.

Holloway, I. & Wheeler, S. (2002) *Qualitative research in nursing*, 2nd Edn. Oxford: Blackwell Publishing.

Hynson, J.L., Aroni, R., Bauld, C. & Sawyer, S.M. (2006) Research with bereaved parents: A question of how not why. *Palliative Medicine* **20**(8), 805–811.

Knafl, K.A. & Deatrick, J.A. (2005) Top 10 tips for successful qualitative grantsmanship. *Research in Nursing & Health*, **28**(6), 441–443.

Letourneau, N. & Allen, M. (1999) Post-positivistic critical multiplism: A beginning dialogue. *Journal of Advanced Nursing* **30**(3), 623–630.

Lincoln, Y.S. & Guba, E.G. (1985) *Naturalistic inquiry.* Newbury Park, CA: Sage.

Mauthner, N.S. & Doucet, H. (2003) Reflexive accounts and accounts of reflexivity in qualitative data analysis. *Sociology* **37**(3), 413–431.

Mead, M. (2001) *Coming of age in Samoa: A psychological study of primitive youth for western civilisation.* New York: HarperCollins.

Miller, F.A. & Alvarado, K. (2005) Incorporating documents into qualitative nursing research. *Journal of Nursing Scholarship* **37**(4), 348–353.

Montgomery, P. & Bailey, P.H. (2007) Field notes and theoretical memos in grounded theory. *Western Journal of Nursing Research* **29**(1), 65–79.

Murphy, F. (2005) Preparing for the field: Developing competence as an ethnographic field worker. *Nurse Researcher* **12**(3), 52–60.

Potter, P.J. & Frisch, N. (2007) Holistic assessment and care: Presence in the process. *Nursing Clinics of North America* **42**(2), 213–228.

Power, E.M. (2004) Toward understanding in postmodern interview analysis: Interpreting the contradictory remarks of a research participant. *Qualitative Health Research* **14**(6), 858–865.

Sandelowski, M. (1993) Rigor or rigor mortis: The problem of rigor in qualitative research revisited. *Advances in Nursing Science* **16**(2), 1–8.

Sandelowski, M. (1998) Writing a good read: Strategies for re-presenting qualitative analysis. *Research in Nursing & Health* **21**(4), 375–382.

Sandelowski, M. (2000) Whatever happened to qualitative description? *Research in Nursing & Health* **23**(4), 334–340.

Sandelowski, M. (2004) Using qualitative research. *Qualitative Health Research* **14**(10), 1366–1386.

Schwartz-Barcott, D., Patterson, B.J., Lusardi, P. & Farmer, B.C. (2002) From practice to theory: Tightening the link via three fieldwork strategies. *Journal of Advanced Nursing* **39**(3), 281–289.

Silverman, D. (2006) *Interpreting qualitative data: Methods for analyzing talk, text and interaction*, 3rd Edn. Thousand Oaks, CA: Sage Publications.

Slaughter, S., Dean, Y., Knight, H., Krieg, B., Mor, P., Nour, V., et al. (2007) The inevitable pull of the river's current: Interpretations derived from a single text using multiple research traditions. *Qualitative Health Research* **17**(4), 548–561.

Tuckett, A.G. (2004) Qualitative research sampling: The very real complexities. *Nurse Researcher* **12**(1), 47–61.

Ungar, M. (2006) 'Too ambitious': What happens when funders misunderstand the strengths of qualitative research design? *Qualitative Social Work* **5**(2), 261–277.

Van Manen, M. (2006) Writing qualitatively, or the demands of writing. *Qualitative Health Research* **16**(5), 713–722.

Vivar, C.G., McQueen, A., Whyte, D.A. & Armayor, N.C. (2007) Getting started with qualitative research: Developing a research proposal. *Nurse Researcher* **14**(3), 60–73.

Weaver, K. & Olson, J.K. (2006) Understanding paradigms used for nursing research. *Journal of Advanced Nursing* **53**(4), 459–469.

Weitzman, E.A. (1999) Analyzing qualitative data with computer software. *Health Services Research* **34**(5), 1241–1263.

Whittemore, R., Chase, S.K. & Mandle, C.L. (2001) Validity in qualitative research. *Qualitative Health Research* **11**(4), 522–537.

Wickham, M. & Woods, M. (2005) Reflecting on the strategic use of CAQDAS to manage and report on the qualitative research process. *Qualitative Report* **10**(4), 687–702.

Willis, J.W. (2007) *Foundations of qualitative research: Interpretive and critical approaches.* Thousand Oaks, CA: Sage Publications.

Wolf, M. (1992) *A thrice told tale: Feminism, postmodernism, and ethnographic responsibility.* Stanford: Stanford University Press.

Wolfinger, N.H. (2002) On writing fieldnotes: Collection strategies and background expectancies. *Qualitative Research* **2**(1), 85–95.

Chapter 16
Preparing qualitative data for analysis

Teri Lindgren

Introduction

Analyzing data from a primary or secondary source is easier and much less time-consuming if researchers first plan how they will gather information and then systematically prepare it for evaluation. Everyone acknowledges that textual documents need to be 'cleaned' for the purpose of accurate analysis, yet few authors explain the data cleaning process. This chapter describes the necessary steps, which include identifying and resolving data problems, and managing, editing, and formatting the information.

Good data preparation is essential, but it cannot compensate for a poor research design or missteps in information gathering. Other chapters in this book discuss proper planning of research to avoid difficulties in data analysis.

Qualitative data arise from interviews, focus groups, field observations, audio or video recordings, and documents. The goals of qualitative data analysis depend somewhat on the study methodology, but, generally, such analysis describes similarities and differences, tells stories about experiences, identifies themes and patterns, summarizes responses, and interprets meanings (Ryan & Bernard 2000). Textual information – transcribed interviews, notes about observations of study participants, and printed materials – is the most common form of qualitative data.

The methodology and its philosophical underpinnings determine the manner of data collection and analysis, and the necessary sample size. For example, phenomenology investigators often conduct in-depth, lengthy, and multiple interviews with a fairly limited number of participants and apply intensive interpretive or narrative analysis. Grounded theory investigators, in contrast, may interview a larger number of people, take extensive observational field notes, examine textual and audiovisual information, and use extensive and evolving coding systems in their analyses.

In any case, before analysis begins, the researcher must consider several issues. One is the volume of data – the number and length of interviews, the kinds of documents to be examined, or the extent of observational notes. A small project, such as a pilot study, is less comprehensive and complex than a larger undertaking; therefore, it offers more flexibility in terms of data preparation. A second issue is the effort and time necessary to transcribe interviews. A third is the data analysis process, which depends on the research design and methodology. Finally, will the investigator use a software program to facilitate the analysis or rely on the more traditional pencil and paper approach?

Collection, transcription, and management

How one collects qualitative data affects data preparation. If the information will come primarily from interviews, an important consideration is how the interviews will be recorded. If the information will come mostly from observational notes, recordings are not necessary. Regardless of the source and manner of collection, data need to be put into a usable form for analysis.

Because qualitative analysis tends to be an iterative process (Hammersley & Atkinson 1995), researchers often modify their semi-structured interview guidelines as participants' initial responses to questions raise new ideas that need to be explored or it becomes apparent that participants do not fully understand some questions. Therefore, quick access to interview transcriptions is key – a factor that figures into plans for recording, transcribing, editing, and formatting information.

Collection

When researchers design a study, they must decide what to record and how. Typically, they record lengthy interviews. However, sometimes this is not possible, perhaps because participants object or the setting does not allow it – for example, when there is too much noise, or when privacy is lacking. In this situation, investigators must be prepared to take extensive notes.

Choosing the right recording device can be an important design decision that ultimately affects data preparation. In the past, researchers used manual tape recorders. However, these machines have a number of limitations. Background noise can make it difficult to hear everything participants said, changing tapes periodically may interrupt the flow of long interviews, and tapes may need to be transported or shipped to a transcriptionist who has the right equipment to transcribe them, including foot pedals to stop, rewind, and restart the tapes.

Because digital recorders present fewer problems; they are more popular. Most are small and unobtrusive, offer good to excellent sound quality (they can filter out ambient noise to some extent), and have a greater storage capacity than manual recorders, precluding interruptions to change tapes. Digital recorders produce audio files that, with the proper software, can be downloaded to a computer or burned on to computer discs. Sending the files electronically to a transcriptionist is much easier than physically carrying or shipping them, and if the transcriptionist has a computer and the right software, no other special equipment is necessary. In the past, digital recorders were expensive; now, there is not a large difference in price between manual and digital recorders, especially when one factors in the tape and transcription equipment costs for manual recorders.

Transcription

Numerous factors affect the manner of transcription. It takes time to type handwritten field notes, but it may take considerably longer to transcribe recordings verbatim, unless the transcriptionist is especially skilled. A researcher must determine who will perform the transcription and, depending on the size of a study, how much time it will take. An advantage of self-transcription in a small study is that the researcher becomes familiar with the data early on, which allows more iterative data collection and analysis. However, the time necessary for self-transcription may outweigh the benefits of immersion in the data. Even a skilled transcriptionist can easily spend 6–8 hours transcribing an hour of recorded interview material.

Larger projects require that the investigator hire or train one or more transcriptionists – people who understand the ethical and confidentiality aspects of research, can transcribe materials verbatim, and can complete the process in a timely fashion. Finding the right transcriptionist may be difficult, but this task is easier when one asks colleagues, acquaintances, and relatives if they know of potential candidates.

Management

Data management involves controlling the data format and maintaining the confidentiality of participants. Researchers must keep data identification numbers and participant identifiers separate. All transcriptions should include an identification number and the date and location of the interview. If there are multiple data collectors and/or transcriptionists, identifying them can be helpful. For confidentiality purposes, transcriptionists need to know what to do with names embedded in interviews.

Another ethical concern is the protection of audiotapes and computer files. Tapes need to be transferred and stored safely (to preserve their quality) and securely (to protect the privacy of interviewees). Only the researchers should have access to computer files, and e-mail must be protected from confidentiality breaches. Research institutions have various confidentiality safeguards, such as locked drawers for tapes and security codes for computers files. Finally, all tapes and files should be destroyed at the end of a study in an effective and ecologically sensitive manner.

Preparing data for analysis

The major part of data preparation is editing and formatting.

Editing

All textual data must be edited for readability, which may reveal transcription errors or questions. Early in the data collection process and with each new transcriptionist, the researcher must compare transcriptions with the recording or notes for accuracy and, if problems emerge, discuss them with the transcriptionist. These reviews can be very time-consuming but once transcription trustworthiness has been established, random spot reviews should be sufficient.

Simple spelling and grammar checks can highlight oddities in the transcription, such as phrases or sentences that do not make sense or incorrect word selection, such as 'their' instead of 'there.' Depending on a study's context, grammar checks should not alter participants' unique language characteristics, word usage, or flow of dialogue, as changes could affect the data analysis. It is acceptable to correct grammar in the written analysis for publication, but preserving the original language as much as possible maintains the connections between the data and the emerging patterns, themes, and concepts. The danger is that the researcher will create, rather than interpret, data.

Working with translated text presents special challenges. For example, a USA-based team of researchers investigating HIV-related messages in Malawi – a small, poor country in southern Africa where most of the study participants did not speak English – hired local people to conduct interviews in Chichewa, the primary language there, and to translate and transcribe the interviews into handwritten form. The researchers then typed up and edited the transcriptions before they left Malawi. This enabled them to question the interviewers about unclear text or English translations that seemed a bit odd. They also hired well-educated and experienced local researchers to help with this verification process.

An issue in such cases is deciding which words should remain in the original language and which should be translated. Many words are culturally unique – there is no equivalent meaning in another language. In the course of collecting data in German, for example, a researcher discovered that certain words carried a broad sense or feeling; trying to capture their true meaning in English would have required lengthy descriptions. Similarly, the researchers in Malawi concluded that literal translations of certain cultural practices would not express what these practices represented in people's lives, and that explaining the culturally embedded norms underlying them would be cumbersome. In both studies, the researchers therefore decided not to translate particular words.

Formatting

The format, or page layout, of textual data depends on how the researcher prefers to read the information and whether he or she will use a computer program. As ideas and patterns emerge over the course of a study, the format may have to be altered.

In paper and pencil analyses, the analysis method is a format consideration. Narrative 'whole read' approaches, such as those in studies of phenomena or discourse, typically analyze interviews by presenting comments and memoranda that explain the entire text. Sociologic and anthropologic approaches, such as those in grounded theory or ethnographic studies, are more likely to break text apart using various types of coding to designate social processes or themes.

For narratives, an easily read format often is best – a 12-point font, double spacing, and margins of 2.5–3 cm. If there will be lots of coding, a better format is a 12-point font, single or double spacing, and a right margin of 7.5–9 cm. Coding entered in the right margin enables the researcher to connect a code visually with the text it demarks.

In either case, it is helpful to clearly distinguish interviewers' questions and comments from participants' responses. Labeling the interviewers 'I' and the respondents 'R,' and leaving extra space between questions and responses in the text, is one way to accomplish this. Ultimately, the researcher's format preferences are the most important factor because they reflect what he or she is most comfortable with visually and what will be most practical in data analysis.

Formats that used computer assisted qualitative data analysis software (CAQDAS) previously required that all files be saved in a text format (.txt) or rich text format (.rtf). The most commonly used software now accepts documents formatted in either Microsoft Word or Word Perfect. However, the software still changes documents to a rich text format, so some formatting, such as bold and highlighted text, may not show up when the researcher reads interviews in the application. Although the investigator's preference in terms of visual and analytical comfort is the most important factor, some pre-testing to see what format works best in a particular software product might be helpful. For example, when reading hard-copy interviews, the authors prefer double spacing, but when they upload documents to their software program, they find that single spacing is more comfortable visually and facilitates analysis.

Manual versus digital analysis techniques

While the size of a study often dictates whether researchers should analyze data manually or digitally, a major consideration is their comfort with one or the other approach. For a pilot study that will yield limited data, cutting and pasting text in a physical document may be preferable. For larger studies, qualitative research software that helps organize and manage data may be better.

Paper and pencil

Qualitative analysis seeks to boil down textual data into patterns, themes, codes, or interpretations. It requires a way to code and then sort the data. For many years, investigators have successfully used a number of inexpensive manual techniques to accomplish this. For example, in the margins of hard-copy interviews, they have made notes or inserted codes to signify particular textual data, then created index cards containing codes and quotes, and sorted the information into distinctive groups based on themes, patterns, and/or concepts. Other investigators have used color-coding schemes to connect codes or themes with exemplary quotes. Still others have attached codes and themes to walls to get a big-picture view of any patterns and relationships that may exist. However, such techniques can become cumbersome and time-consuming when there are analytical teams or large data sets.

Digital tools

Computers and software have transformed qualitative analysis. Although tensions surround the use of technology for this purpose (Seale 2005), experienced researchers increasingly rely on word processing software and/or CAQDAS to help them manipulate, reduce, and interpret data sets that are large, complex, or both. Word processing software is the simplest tool; it enables researchers to search for keywords or strings of text, which aids coding, text retrieval, and count analysis. Judicious highlighting of text can replace color-coding schemes, and creating thematic files can help sort codes and quotes. Cutting and pasting text in digital files is very easy.

As the level of abstraction increases during analysis, the researcher must maintain the connection between a concept or theme and the data, such as quotes, from which it is derived. One way to track these links in a word processing application is to format textual materials using numbered lines, and, in the analysis, to note the origin of information about a concept or theme – for example, 'Interview #2, lines 35–40.'

CAQDAS became available in the mid-1980s and proliferated in the 1990s. Qualitative researchers cited the potential usefulness of CAQDAS, especially the speed of text demarcation with coding and complex networking of interpretations (Weitzman 1999). Articles comparing the various CAQDAS applications in research also proliferated. Now, many types of this software are on the market.[1]

Extensive discussion about CAQDAS in the literature revealed the usefulness of certain applications for particular qualitative methodologies, including grounded theory. Heeding these discussions, CAQDAS producers continually upgraded their programs to fix problems. The unchallenged assumption was that CAQDAS would automatically improve qualitative research by increasing rigor and validity, and by identifying new ways to analyze data (St. John & Johnson 2000; McMillan & Koenig 2004; Seale 2005). Consequently, some viewed CAQDAS as a click-of-the-mouse solution, failing to understand that it is only an analysis aid (Jennings 2007; Sandelowski & Barroso 2007).

Finding and choosing the right CAQDAS application is not quick or easy.[2] Weitzman (1999) identified five families of software programs, although only three were developed specifically to assist with qualitative data analysis. One family of applications is code-and-retrieve programs, such as Ethnograph, HyperQual 2, and QualPro, which enable researchers to demark or code pieces of text as quotes and display all quotes associated with a code. The second family, code-based theory builders, allow representation of relationships among codes and/or hierarchical ordering of them. These applications include NVivo, NUD*ST, and ATLAS.ti. The third family is conceptual network builders. They perform like theory builders but have an additional feature; graphic representation of relationships among codes and concepts in networks. This facilitates greater abstraction and the grounding of interpretation in data (Weitzman 1999).

Answering key questions can help a researcher decide which CAQDAS program is appropriate:

- What type of data will be collected? Some software packages are better suited for parsing audio or visual data, while others are designed for textual data. A potentially important factor regarding software for textual data is whether it supports all of the languages a researcher needs. Some programs can only handle Latinized scripts, which will pose difficulties if one is trying to analyze interviews in languages that use different characters, such as Mandarin, Korean, Russian, or Arabic.

- Will data be collected from one source or from multiple sources that may require comparisons within and among groups? For example, if a researcher plans to study the impact of the loss of a family member, will he or she collect data only from mothers (one level) or from mothers, fathers, and children (three levels)? If the latter, he or she might consider using a program that enables him or her to look at the data from one family or from one of the three levels, perhaps children.

- What kind of analysis will be performed? If an analysis requires that text be coded and that the codes be exported to a manuscript, any of the common CAQDAS applications would work. If, however, the researcher wants to develop theory by creating conceptual hierarchies or patterns, a code-based theory builder would be more useful.

- Will a team of researchers analyze the data? The team approach requires a program to facilitate this task. For example, ATLAS.ti allows multiple investigators to code the same data simultaneously and independently, then merge their coded information into one data set for further refinement by the team.

- Does a CAQDAS application's visual presentation of text and codes meet the researcher's analytical needs? One way to find out is to test the software on a trial basis. Ethnograph, one of the oldest programs, and NUD*ST were designed for ethnographic research and grounded theory research, respectively, so neither may be the best choice for the particular type of study an investigator has in mind. Although the major vendors claim that their qualitative software programs are useful in all qualitative research, the terminology these products use – for example, for types of documents, codes, memos, quotations, field notes – often reflects a certain qualitative methodology. The wise researcher is one who makes sure that his or her understanding of the terms an application uses is consistent with programmers' interpretation. For example, qualitative researchers often write memos containing thoughts about data, codes and their meanings, decisions made during data analysis, relationships between data, and theoretical ideas. A number of applications have a memo function, but programmers and researchers may conceptualize this function differently.

- Are data documents stored in the application or elsewhere? ATLAS.ti does not store interviews or observational notes; rather, it identifies the pathway to a document and returns to the pathway when it seeks that document for viewing. This function includes requirements for document storage and formatting. Documents assigned to ATLAS.ti cannot be moved to a different location on the computer, and those located elsewhere cannot be found. The analytical program and documents must always travel together in the same file, otherwise information could be lost. Furthermore, changing a document that has already been assigned will also disconnect it from the program. For example, despite good editing of transcribed documents, some small or even large errors inevitably appear during data analysis. The temptation is to fix errors. However, the program does not 'see' a fixed document because it is

not the one previously assigned, so all work in the revised document will be lost. Knowing in advance how an application connects to data will preclude problems later on.
- What computer skills does the researcher have? Novices may be taking on more than they can handle by choosing a CAQDAS application, and even skilled investigators might discover that the learning curve is too steep. Can they devote enough time to becoming familiar with the software? Is technical support available from one or more sources? Glitches or improper use of the application could jeopardize all of the time and effort the researcher has spent collecting, formatting, and analyzing data.

Conclusions

Steps in preparing textual data for qualitative studies include collection, transcription, management, editing, and formatting. Investigators can analyze data manually, with traditional paper and pencil techniques, or digitally, using qualitative research software, which may be better for larger studies. They should ask key questions when seeking a software product that will meet their needs.

Notes

1 The American Evaluation Association has an extensive list of CAQDAS products at www.eval.org/Resources/QDA.htm.
2 See caqdas.soc.surrey.ac.uk/ChoosingLewins&SilverV5July06.pdf for summaries of the most commonly used CAQDAS applications. Some products are available for free trials. They include NVivo and NUD*ST (www.qsrinternational.com/products_previous-products_n6.aspx), ATLAS.ti (www.atlasti.com), and Ethnograph (www.qualisresearch.com).

References

Hammersley, M. & Atkinson, P. (1995) *Ethnography*, 2nd Edn. London: Routledge.
Jennings, B.M. (2007) Qualitative analysis: A case of software or 'peopleware'? *Research in Nursing and Health* **30**(5), 483–484.
MacMillan, K. & Koenig, T. (2004) The wow factor: Preconceptions and expectations for data analysis software in qualitative research. *Social Science Computer Review* **22**(2), 179–186.
Ryan, G.W. & Bernard, H.R. (2000) Data management and analysis methods. In N.K. Denzin & Y.S. Lincoln (Eds) *Handbook of qualitative research*, 2nd Edn. Thousand Oaks, CA: Sage Publications.
Sandelowski, M. & Barroso, J. (2007) *Handbook for synthesizing qualitative research.* New York: Springer Publishing.
Seale, C. (2005) Using computers to analyse qualitative data. In D. Silverman (Ed) *Doing qualitative research*. London: Sage Publications.
St. John, W. & Johnson, P. (2000) The pros and cons of data analysis software for qualitative research. *Journal of Nursing Scholarship* **32**(4), 393–397.
Weitzman, E.A. (1999) Analyzing qualitative data with computer software. *Health Services Research* **34**(5 Pt 2), 1241–1263.

Part 5
Research ethics

Chapter 17
Responsible conduct of research

William L. Holzemer

Ethics in nursing research and practice

The International Council of Nurses (ICN) has provided leadership for nursing- and health care-related ethical issues since its founding in 1899. In 1953, the Council of National Representatives adopted the first international code of nursing ethics. The ICN's *Code of Ethics for Nurses*, revised in 2006, is still disseminated worldwide.

As medical and scientific technology advance, individuals and society face complex dilemmas and difficult bioethical issues, such as extending life, preserving the quality of life, treating terminal illnesses, conducting stem cell and other experimental research, and altering the human genome. Fry and Johnstone (2006) cited three themes that have focused greater attention on the responsible conduct of research: the growth of the field of medical ethics; the rapid expansion of systematic experimentation; and policy development, which is linking the explosion of knowledge to clinical practice guidelines and funding mechanisms. Today, bioethics is an extremely important area of ethics.[1]

The ICN's definition of nursing is at the foundation of bioethical issues in nursing research:

> Nursing encompasses autonomous and collaborative care of individuals of all ages, families, groups and communities, sick or well and in all settings. Nursing includes the promotion of health, prevention of illness, and the care of ill, disabled, and dying people. Advocacy, promotion of a safe environment,

research, participating in shaping health policy and in patient and health systems management, and education are also key nursing roles.[2]

The ICN *Code of Ethics for Nurses* (ICN 2006) affirms that nurses play a major part in conducting research that will build evidence for practice. It provides a foundation for all nursing roles, including those of clinician, teacher, manager, and researcher. Nursing ethics, or norms for conduct that distinguish between acceptable and unacceptable behavior, include respecting the dignity of, and providing collaborative care to, patients. Research ethics promote the aims of research and ensure accountability to the public. They lead to an understanding of acceptable and unacceptable behaviors in research and to discussions about scientific integrity.

Scientific integrity

A high standard of scientific integrity is necessary to avoid misconduct in research. At a minimum, the scientific community and the public expect adherence to standards of intellectual honesty in the formulation, conduct, review, and reporting of studies.

The Nuremberg Code (Mitscherlich & Mielke 1949), the Declaration of Helsinki (Human & Fluss 2001), and the Belmont Report: Ethical Principles and Guidelines for the Protection of Human Subjects of Research (Department of Health, Education, and Welfare 1979)[3] constitute the foundation for scientific integrity and the protection of research participants. The Nuremberg Code grew out of the devastating human 'research' conducted during World War II without any concept of voluntary participation or consent. The Declaration of Helsinki fostered better understanding of the differences between therapeutic and non-therapeutic research, and of the kinds of information that potential research subjects must receive. The Belmont Report, which the US government published in response to unethical behavior in research (Karigan 2001), cites specific ethical problems in studies on humans and focuses on protecting patients from unethical investigators.

Shamoo and Resnik (2003) outlined 15 ethical principles in the conduct of research (Table 17.1). Because nursing research often involves patients, there is an element of human rights vulnerability. Vulnerability refers to a power relationship wherein a person is at risk for something because he or she has less stature, income, or education than another person does, or has different characteristics. Inpatients are vulnerable because decisions may be made for them without their knowledge or consent. Inpatients and outpatients are also vulnerable when they cannot make volitional or voluntary decisions about participating in an experimental procedure or research.[4] Vulnerability in research subjects refers to the potential harms and risks versus the potential benefits of participation. Among potential subjects, this is complicated by the fact that some patients may feel obligated to participate because they receive care in that setting.

All patients, by definition, are considered to be vulnerable, given that they are in a care environment. However, some individuals or groups are more vulnerable than others. Examples include comatose patients and newborn infants, as they cannot participate in decision-making regarding their care nor

Table 17.1 Principles for ethical conduct of research.

Principles	Definitions
Honesty	Being truthful in all aspects of research
Objectivity	Avoiding bias in communication, design, analysis, and reporting
Integrity	Keeping promises and agreements, particularly with colleagues and research participants
Carefulness	Avoiding carelessness and keeping good records
Openness	Sharing data/results and being open to critique
Respect for intellectual property	Honoring copyrighted materials, patents, etc., and not using other researchers' work without permission
Confidentiality	Protecting all research-related documents, including grant applications, manuscripts in review, and patient data
Responsible publication	Publishing to build knowledge and sharing results
Education	Educating and mentoring future research scientists
Respect for colleagues	Treating colleagues, students, and research participants fairly
Social responsibility	Being responsible to communities and promoting social good
Non-discrimination	Avoiding discrimination related to sex, race, ethnicity, sexual orientation, and other factors
Competence	Maintaining professional competence
Legality	Knowing and abiding by relevant laws and regulations
Animal care	Respecting animals by adhering to international standards of care
Human subjects protection	Minimizing harms and risks to, and maximizing benefits for, research participants

give informed consent to participate in research. Patients who do not speak the primary language of a care setting are particularly vulnerable (Ledger 2002).

Prospective study subjects are vulnerable when they may not feel free to decline if an authoritative person favors their participation. Vulnerable groups, such as school children or prisoners, are confined; they may feel obligated to participate in a study or experiment because a teacher or prison guard informed them about the research. The special needs of vulnerable groups must be considered in discussions about how to protect the rights of potential subjects.

Six ethical principles guide the protection of prospective research participants: beneficence, non-maleficence, fidelity, justice, veracity, and confidentiality.

Beneficence means doing good for the research participant and society. It includes the benefit of participating in a study, such as access to regular health care in an ongoing clinical trial or access to experimental therapies (Spencer 1997). Researchers should ask themselves: What good will study participants receive?

Non-maleficence means doing no harm to research participants. Researchers should ask themselves: What harm might come to those who agree to participate in this study? The potential risks must be articulated, written down, and discussed with prospective subjects.

Fidelity means creating trust between the investigator and participant. Researchers should assess how they will build trust with their subjects over time.

There are classic examples of studies that demonstrated a total lack of fidelity. The most famous case in the USA was a natural history study of syphilis among African-American men in Tuskegee, Alabama, who participated without their knowledge or consent. When a syphilis therapy became available, participants were not informed (Jones 1993).

Justice means being fair to participants and not providing differential support to one or another group. It is intimately linked with fidelity and veracity.

Veracity means telling the truth to study participants. Investigators are ethically responsible for being honest with subjects and informing them of all known potential risks and benefits. Cultures vary in terms of the amount of information patients receive regarding their diagnoses and treatments. Consequently, it may be a challenge to construct a consent form for patients who have not been informed of their diagnosis. The investigator must determine, depending on the proposed study, how important it is to do so. The consent form might only need to state, 'You are being asked to participate in a study because you are ill,' rather than, 'You are being asked to participate in a study because you have cancer.' Investigators are ethically obliged to consider veracity within the context of culture.

Confidentiality means safeguarding personal information collected during a study and making sure others do not see it, usually by never reporting an individual's data. Maintaining confidentiality is different from ensuring anonymity. If a researcher is conducting interviews, data collection cannot be anonymous, as the investigator has met the participants. Nor can medical records be anonymous. However, the confidentiality of aggregate data can and must be protected.

To ensure scientific integrity, nurse scientists need to be trained in the responsible conduct of research.

Responsible conduct of research

Data accuracy and integrity

Research data are all types of records, protocols, procedures, and results collected or reviewed in a study. Everyone involved in the research is responsible for data accuracy and integrity. The National Institutes of Health in the USA recommends that researchers keep data for 5 years before destroying them in case there are any questions about the accuracy of published results or if someone wants to reanalyze the information. The principal investigator is responsible for developing, maintaining, and managing study findings with the utmost organization to protect participants' rights and to enable future access to specific data.

Ethical guidelines for conducting research are related to the rigor of science itself. In quantitative research, investigators control for potential bias by selecting the design and by using valid and reliable measures and the appropriate level of analysis, based on the type of data they collect. Investigators are responsible for understanding the concept of bias and how it relates to their particular study design.

Careful data management – storage, retrieval, and ownership – is necessary so bias is not introduced. Work environments may have different rules about archiving data; the investigator must know these rules and follow them. In quantitative research, other investigators might try to replicate results from a previously published study by checking the coding of an item and reanalyzing the data, as decisions about how data are coded can influence findings.

Ethical conduct includes the capability to share research materials with other investigators at appropriate times. Researchers may receive requests to provide raw data for additional analysis, such as a meta-analysis, which evaluates data from multiple published studies. A data code book allows relatively easy interpretation several years after a study has been completed. Investigators in the laboratory sciences use a notebook to track their thinking and actions over time, while other types of researchers rarely document every step so precisely. In long-running projects, note-taking makes it easier to reconstruct the rationale investigators used to make a series of decisions.

Publication and authorship

Scientists are responsible for completing their research. The last step is disseminating and publishing the results so the scientific community can assess, review, validate, and build upon them.

There are different authorship models and philosophies, which are beyond the scope of this chapter, but, in general, the scientific community agrees that authors need to have made a significant contribution to the conceptualization, design, execution, and interpretation of a study, and must be willing to assume responsibility for it. Novices who start out by working as a research assistant or data clerk would not expect to be listed as an author. However, if someone contributes to project development, has an impact on data collection procedures, helps analyze data, and writes parts of the manuscript, it is probably appropriate to raise the issue of listing that person as an author. Most importantly, authorship and the order of authors on a manuscript should be discussed before it is written, an easy task if communication among research team members is open and honest.

'Gift' authorship – for example, citing the name of the laboratory director or program chairperson, in deference to their professional status – is inappropriate unless that individual had a substantial impact on the study's scientific direction. Distinguished scientists have been publicly embarrassed when challenged about published papers that bore their name even though they knew very little about the research.

Usually, the order of authors on a paper signifies the degree of their participation, with the first author having made the largest contribution. Credit should also be given to other investigators for research they have carried out on the same or related topic. If a researcher conducts a study that builds on his or her earlier work, that work should be cited too, because it enables readers to track the investigator's research over time. This also discourages authors from publishing the same data in different journals. A clear synthesis of published research, with appropriate references, is the best way to credit prior work.

Even if research yields a potential breakthrough, seasoned scientists oppose premature publication, preferring instead to wait until they or others have replicated – and thus confirmed – the findings. They also avoid using television, newspapers, or other media as the first outlet for reporting results, a tactic the scientific community frowns upon because the findings have not undergone peer review. Once an article has been published in a peer-reviewed journal, interviews with the popular press may be quite appropriate.

Ethical researchers refrain from plagiarizing ideas and words (Vogelsang 1997). This includes not reciting significant sections of one's own previously published work. Today, computer software and the Internet make it quite easy to detect plagiarism, which often results from miscommunication among scientists or pressure to produce information quickly. Good communication among scientists, and methods to prevent early publication of findings, help inhibit plagiarism.

Another ethical obligation is to report sufficient information so another investigator can replicate the findings. Replication generally makes good sense in quantitative research; how it applies to qualitative studies is less clear. All research methods include standards for rigor that specify the types of information investigators should report. Authors must know these standards.

Peer review

Peer review is critical evaluation of scientific work before publication. Responsible science relies on peer review – research funding and everyday decisions about whether or not manuscripts warrant publication are based on it. Professionals who critique a study must understand that all materials are privileged and should not be shared with others.

There is a potential conflict of interest if someone who is asked to review a draft manuscript or grant application has a relationship with the author, works at the same institution, or has been a mentor for the grant applicant. Declining to participate, which is customary in such cases, ensures there is neither a perceived nor real conflict of interest (Gopee 2001).

Safeguards for potential conflict of interest include knowledge, objectivity, and impartiality. Scientists who review proposals, manuscripts, or grant applications must be as knowledgeable and up-to-date as possible about their area of expertise in order to provide an unbiased evaluation. Objectivity is a hallmark of research. While some authors question the objectivity of peer review (Martin 1986), it is a primary mechanism for controlling bias. The best protection against conflicts of interest and bias is to have multiple experts simultaneously review a study proposal or manuscript, and render an objective, independent, and honest opinion of its significance and technical merit.

Touretzky (1998) cited 10 responsibilities of peer reviewers:

(1) Prospective reviewers should agree to do a review if asked;
(2) If a manuscript or grant application is outside of the prospective reviewer's area of expertise or there is a perceived conflict of interest, the manuscript or application should be returned promptly;
(3) Reviewers should judge the quality of a manuscript objectively;
(4) Reviewers should avoid potential conflicts of interest;
(5) A personal or professional relationship with the author, such as a student, precludes participation in a review;
(6) Manuscripts should remain confidential;
(7) Citations should accompany the reviewer's judgments;

(8)   If a reviewer knows the literature well, he or she should note missing citations;

(9)   All reviews should be promptly returned; and

(10) Reviewers should not use ideas from manuscripts or grant applications in their own work.

Novice nurse scientists can learn about peer review by critiquing colleagues' work. As scientists' careers advance, there is a greater expectation that they will donate time and energy to peer reviews.

Mentor–trainee relationships

A successful mentoring relationship is one in which the trainee gains sound skills in conducting research and attaining career goals (Byrne & Keefe 2002). Mentorship is an essential obligation of senior scientists. It should foster freedom for the mentee to pursue scientific inquiry, critical evaluation, and personal and professional integrity and growth.

Although mentorship is perhaps the essence of graduate education, it also poses potential conflict risks (Fawcett 2002). When faculty members work closely with graduate students over time, ownership of ideas may become blurred during many hours of dialogue, data interpretation, and project planning. Sometimes it would be easier to simply exclude students from these opportunities, yet true mentorship may occur during such interactions. There is no simple solution to this dilemma. Therefore, periodic assessment of potential conflicts and open, honest communication are extremely important.

Faculty mentors have an ethical responsibility not only to teach and support students, but also to give them appropriate credit. In addition, they are obligated to teach the responsible conduct of research (Blair & Schaffer 1991). Mentees have the right to find a new mentor if they believe that the relationship does not support their career goals or intellectual freedom.

Multidisciplinary research teams

Research on health and illness topics often requires interdisciplinary or multidisciplinary teams to build a sound research plan for testing an intervention or answering a particular question. For example, a geneticist might join a nurse scientist in examining the biomarkers of symptoms.

Effective collaboration often necessitates ground rules or operational procedures. Collaborators must discuss and agree on issues such as individual responsibilities, ownership of data, rights to published data, authorship, and the order of authors on a manuscript for publication.

Protection of human and animal subjects

The use of humans and animals in research is essential to improving human health, but it requires compliance with ethical and legal guidelines. Obtaining informed consent is both a legal and moral obligation. Institutional review boards (IRBs) must approve all human and animal research and must be informed of any related circumstances. Investigators need training in the protection of human research subjects – the focus of most nursing research – or animal welfare.

Four ethical principles guide research involving human subjects: the right not to be harmed; the right to full disclosure; the right of self-determination; and the right of privacy, confidentiality, and anonymity.

Sometimes there are negative side effects in biomedical intervention studies, especially drug-related research. If the risk is extremely high, such a study may not be warranted. In all cases, participants have the right not to be harmed.

The right of full disclosure means research subjects should be informed about any and all risks and benefits. It is unethical to withhold information that might affect a potential subject's decision about whether to participate. Researchers who conduct randomized controlled trials must tell participants they may be assigned to one or another treatment, or perhaps to no treatment, even if an individual prefers a certain therapy. Investigators may not always achieve full disclosure, particularly if they do not perceive a potential risk or benefit (Higgins & Daly 2002).

After full disclosure, prospective research subjects have the right to freely determine for themselves if they want to participate. The right of self-determination assumes there is no coercion, which can arise when researchers offer a significant financial incentive to low-income individuals or take advantage of vulnerable groups such as children, hospitalized patients, or prisoners. Potential subjects' decision must not have any impact on the regular health care they receive.

If, after giving consent, research subjects feel uncomfortable about the personal nature of questions asked, the right of privacy means they can refuse to answer any of them. Participants also have the right to absolute confidentiality of any information they share with researchers and the right of anonymity, or having their names disassociated from personal data (Meier 2002).

These four ethical principles assume that prospective subjects have sufficient mental capacity and information to make independent decisions. Vulnerable groups may need additional protection, such as child assent and parental consent (Veach et al. 2001). A series of European studies examined this issue in greater detail (Leino-Kilpi et al. 2003; Scott et al. 2003a, 2003b).

Institutional review boards

Most universities and many hospitals and clinics have IRBs or research ethics committees to review proposals for research involving human subjects. These entities seek to prevent harm or injury to participants. Although such reviews are becoming mandatory, in developing countries research ethics committees often do not exist or they have inadequate resources. When they do exist, they may lack independence and expertise (Nuffield Council on Bioethics 2002).

IRB membership should be multidisciplinary in order to ensure expertise in and sensitivity to a broad range of scientific and ethical issues. The boards must take special care to protect the interests of women and other vulnerable populations (Nuffield Council on Bioethics 2002).

According to most guidelines, an IRB may approve research only after the board has determined that a proposed study has met all six of the following requirements:

(1) Risks to subjects will be minimized by procedures that are consistent with sound research design and do not unnecessarily expose subjects to risk;

(2) Risks are reasonable relative to anticipated benefits, if any, and to the importance of the knowledge that one might reasonably expect a study to generate;
(3) Participant selection will be equitable;
(4) Researchers will seek informed consent from each prospective subject or the subject's legally authorized representative, generally by means of a written document;
(5) The research plan makes adequate provisions for ensuring participants' safety; and
(6) There are adequate provisions to protect the privacy of subjects and maintain the confidentiality of data (World Health Organization 2000; Council for International Organizations of Medical Sciences 2002).

Informed consent

Informed consent is the cornerstone of ethically sound research. Participants must have an opportunity to make decisions, without duress, based on complete information. Ethical, legal, and scientific principles guide this process.

The Belmont Report (Department of Health, Education, and Welfare 1979) outlines the ethical principles – information, comprehension, and voluntariness – related to informed consent. Potential research subjects must receive complete information on the research protocol in a form they can comprehend (comprehension is often difficult to judge, given cultural, language, and literacy differences) and they must have a true perception or feeling that their participation is voluntary.

The related legal principles vary by country and sometimes by region within a country. Every researcher is responsible for knowing the legal aspects of gaining informed consent in the country, region, or setting where a study will take place. Sometimes nurse investigators find themselves practicing in a vacuum where it is difficult to obtain guidance regarding the rules of informed consent. In places where there is no informed consent structure because little research has been conducted, nurse scientists can take a leadership role in creating a research ethics committee to ensure adherence to the ethical principles described above. When a country or setting does not have formal informed consent procedures, nurse researchers are ethically obliged to establish them.

Several scientific principles figure into informed consent. Researchers must be experts in their field so they fully understand the potential risks and benefits of study participation. For example, moderate exercise may increase shortness of breath in a patient who has chronic lung disease, but it may also help the patient build lung capacity. An expert in research methods, unlike an expert clinician, might not have sufficient health knowledge to understand the potential risks and benefits.

In addition, investigators should have an excellent understanding of the health care setting so they can identify any coercion to participate in a study, such as a financial reward. Participants might view a modest payment as an acceptable thank-you but an excessive payment as coercive. Other kinds of coercion are more subtle. An example would be a study at a well-child clinic where the average waiting time is 2 hours and study participants need not wait because they receive fixed appointment times to keep the data collectors on schedule.

Often, deferred consent, a subset of informed consent, is necessary when a prospective subject cannot provide informed consent. For example, some countries prohibit informed consent from minors (younger than 18 years old); they require parental consent as well as the minor's verbal assent. Deferred consent also may be necessary from the guardians of mentally or cognitively impaired individuals and critically ill patients, who frequently are unable to provide informed consent. Committees that review requests for approval of human subject research analyze the requests very carefully to ensure that the rights of subjects are protected to the highest degree possible and that the benefits outweigh the risks.

Researchers violate informed consent when they do not obtain consent or when a consenting patient is either not fully informed of study details or is not continually informed of study changes or results.

Informed consent usually involves two stages. First, a research proposal describing the sample instruments, consent forms, and procedures is submitted to an IRB, a process that can be very formal in many countries but nonexistent in others. If there is no IRB, the nurse researcher may lead efforts to create one that comprises expert clinicians, interdisciplinary representatives, research method experts, and community leaders. The IRB basically answers two questions. Has the investigator followed the ethical principles required for informed consent? Do the potential benefits in a proposed study outweigh the potential risks? If the answer to both is yes, the researcher typically can begin approaching potential subjects to obtain informed consent.[5]

In the second stage, investigators gauge prospective subjects' interest in participating by inviting them to learn about the study. If a person agrees, he or she must then carefully read and sign a form titled Consent to Be a Study Participant; the individual receives a copy and the investigator keeps the original. The consent form should indicate how participants can contact the investigator(s) if they have additional questions or concerns. It should also give them the right to terminate participation at any time without any threat to their health or the standard care they otherwise receive.

In some instances, such as research involving illiterate people, a written consent form may be inappropriate, in which case genuine consent must be obtained verbally and include a witness to the consent (Nuffield Council on Bioethics 2002).

The experimental subject's bill of rights

Everyone who is asked to participate in research has the following rights:

- To be told what the study is trying to learn;
- To be told what will happen and if any of the procedures, drugs, or devices are different from those in standard practice;
- To be told about a study's frequent and/or important risks, side effects, or discomforts;
- To be told if they can expect any benefit from participating, and if so, what the benefit might be;
- To be told about other treatment choices and how these may be better or worse than those being studied;
- To be allowed to ask any questions about the study before they agree to participate and during the study;
- To be told what sort of medical treatment is available if any complications arise;

- To have the option not to participate or to drop out after the study has started. This decision should not affect individuals' right to receive the health care they normally would receive;
- To receive a copy of the signed and dated consent form; and
- To be free of pressure when considering whether to participate in the study.[6]

Study subjects often receive a copy of this 'bill of rights' along with an informed consent form.

IRBs request that investigators monitor research participants for adverse events, defined as any unfavorable and unintended sign, symptom, or disease temporarily associated with a medical treatment or procedure regardless of whether it is considered related to a standard medical treatment or procedure that is part of the study. The study's principal investigator is responsible for reporting adverse events to the research team and related institutional bodies. Severe, life-threatening, or fatal adverse events are to be reported within 48 hours of the occurrence. Team members must be trained to recognize, respond to, and record adverse events when or immediately after they occur to ensure the safety of participants. Investigators have an ethical duty to care for those who may suffer adverse effects arising from research (Nuffield Council on Bioethics 2002).

Conflict of interest

An earlier section discussed conflict of interest related to peer review. Conflict of interest, which may be difficult to recognize, also can occur when a person exploits his or her position for personal gain or profit. Researchers are obligated to disclose all relevant relationships, both financial and personal.

There are three types of conflict of interest in science: financial, employment-related, and professional (National Academy of Sciences 1992, 1993). As researchers at a growing number of biotechnology companies splice genes, develop vaccines, and conduct other studies that could lead to lucrative innovations, a conflict of interest may arise in terms of personal financial gain (Castledine 2001; Stokamer 2003). Owning stock in a company that might benefit from research is a classic example of financial conflict of interest. It also is not appropriate if a company consultant reviews an application for a grant the company may receive. Although few nurse scientists have been intimately linked to potential financial gains from research, they need to be aware of these hazards.

Employment-related conflicts of interest (Salvi 2003) are common and easy to spot. For example, if someone is participating with others in a review of grant applications, it is not appropriate for him or her to review applications related to his or her university or place of employment. The individual should leave the room before the application review begins.

A conflict also could arise if a journal asked someone to review a manuscript submitted by a colleague who works at the same institution. Even if the author's name has been stricken from the manuscript, in keeping with a 'blind' review, it is often possible to identify the author based on how the article was written and the literature he or she cited (Callaham 2003). In such cases, prospective reviewers should disqualify themselves.

Professional conflicts of interest can occur when a person's job orientation may interfere with objectivity. An example would be a nurse practitioner who reviews a study examining the impact of care provided by nurse practitioners versus physician assistants. The reviewer may not sense a conflict even though one exists. Gauging the potential for a conflict of interest usually involves self-assessment – asking if one's own expertise, professional affiliations or position, or special knowledge could in any way bias an otherwise objective, fair review of a manuscript or grant application. If the answer is yes, the reviewer should decline to participate.

Misconduct

Conflicts of interest are one of many different kinds of misconduct in research. Others relate to mentorship – for example, mentors who express gender or racial bias, claim mentees' research ideas as their own, or exploit mentees for their own purposes. Teachers have an obligation not only to understand misconduct issues, but to treat their students in an ethical and uncompromising way. In addition, faculties have an obligation to include scientific misconduct in their curricula.

'Whistle blower' refers to someone who makes a claim of misconduct in science. Nurse researchers are responsible for reporting misconduct when they can support their claim with sufficient information or personal knowledge.

Conclusions

Nurse scientists, like other investigators, are obligated to abide by ethical principles when they conduct research. Among the many research issues with ethical implications are data accuracy and integrity, the publication of findings, authorship, peer review, mentor/trainee relationships, protection of human and animal subjects, informed consent, and conflicts of interest.

As in nursing practice, familiarity with the ethics of scientific inquiry is essential. Many universities and other sources offer online training in the protection of human subjects, and some grantmakers, before they even consider grant applications, now require that principal investigators first document such training. Most professional journals will not publish a manuscript without a statement from an institutional review board indicating it approved the study.

All nurses have an ethical responsibility to ensure the protection of patients. In many cases, nurses need to obtain patients' consent before participation in a study, without any coercion, and articulate the risks and benefits. This is a solemn responsibility that should not be taken lightly. When nurses see an absence of appropriate consent procedures for experimental procedures, they are obligated as professionals to speak out on behalf of patients and report this circumstance to appropriate authorities. Patients have a right not be harmed, the right to full disclosure, the right of self-determination, and the right of privacy, confidentiality, and anonymity. Patients trust that nurses will ensure these rights. It is nurses' duty to warrant this trust.

Notes

1 A good resource for understanding the breadth and depth of bioethics is bioethics.od.nih.gov. See also Fry and Johnstone (2006).

2 From www.icn.ch/definition.htm.
3 Available at www.hhs.gov/ohrp/humansubjects/guidance/belmont.htm.
4 Dean and McClement (2002) discuss patients' vulnerability in palliative care.
5 Stevens and Pietsch (2002) discuss issues related to the lack of informed consent for research on women in clinical trials.
6 A version of the bill of rights used by researchers at the University of California, San Francisco, is available at www.research.ucsf.edu/CHR/Guide/chrB_BoR.asp.

References

Blair, C. & Schaffer, W. (1991) Promotion of the responsible conduct of research. *NIH Peer Review Notes* June, 4–6.

Byrne, M.W. & Keefe, M.R. (2002) Building research competence in nursing through mentoring. *Journal of Nursing Scholarship* **34**(4), 391–396.

Callaham, M.L. (2003) Journal policy on ethics in scientific publication. *Annals of Emergency Medicine* **41**(1), 82–89.

Castledine, G. (2001) Case 43: Exploiting nursing status. Nursing home owner who used her nurse status to make business. *British Journal of Nursing* **10**(4), 218.

Council for International Organizations of Medical Sciences (2002) *International ethical guidelines for biomedical research involving human subjects.* Geneva: Council for International Organizations of Medical Sciences.

Dean, R.A. & McClement, S.E. (2002) Palliative care research: Methodological and ethical challenges. *International Journal of Palliative Nursing* **8**(8), 376–380.

Department of Health, Education, and Welfare (1979) *Belmont Report. Ethical principles and guidelines for the protection of human subjects of research.* Washington, D.C.: Department of Health, Education, and Welfare.

Fawcett, D.L. (2002) Mentoring – what it is and how to make it work. *Association of Operating Room Nurses Journal* **75**(5), 950–954.

Fry, S. & Johnstone, M.J. (2006) *Ethics in nursing practice: A guide to ethical decision making,* 3rd Edn. Geneva: International Council of Nurses.

Gopee, N. (2001) The role of peer assessment and peer review in nursing. *British Journal of Nursing* **10**(2), 115–121.

Higgins, P.A. & Daly, B.J. (2002) Knowledge and beliefs of nurse researchers about informed consent principles and regulations. *Nursing Ethics* **9**(6), 663–671.

Human, D. & Fluss, S. (2001) *The World Medical Association's Declaration of Helsinki: Historical and contemporary perspectives,* 5th Draft. Geneva: World Medical Association.

International Council of Nurses (ICN) (2006). *The ICN code of ethics for nurses.* Geneva: International Council of Nurses.

Jones, J.H. (1993) *Bad blood: The Tuskagee syphilis experiment.* New York: Free Press.

Karigan, M. (2001) Ethics in clinical research. *American Journal of Nursing* **101**(9), 26–31.

Ledger, S.D. (2002) Reflections on communicating with non-English-speaking patients. *British Journal of Nursing* **11**(11), 773–780.

Leino-Kilpi, H., Välimäki, M., Dassen, T., Gasull, M., Lemonidou, C., Schopp, A., et al. (2003) Perceptions of autonomy, privacy and informed consent in elderly care in five European countries: General overview. *Nursing Ethics* **10**(1), 18–27.

Martin, B. (1986) Bias in awarding research grants. *British Medical Journal* **293**(6546), 550–552.

Meier, E. (2002) Medical privacy and its value for patients. *Seminars in Oncology Nursing* **18**(2), 105–108.

Mitscherlich, A. & Mielke, F. (1949) The Nuremberg Code (1947). In A. Mitscherlich & F. Mielke (Eds) *Doctors of infamy: The story of the Nazi medical crimes.* New York: Schuman.

National Academy of Sciences Panel on Scientific Responsibility and the Conduct of Research (1992) *Responsible science: Ensuring the integrity of the research process,* Volume 1. Washington, D.C.: National Academy Press.

National Academy of Sciences Panel on Scientific Responsibility and the Conduct of Research (1993) *Responsible science: Ensuring the integrity of the research process,* Volume 2. Washington, D.C.: National Academy Press.

Nuffield Council on Bioethics (2002) *The ethics of research related to healthcare in developing countries.* Plymouth, Devon: Nuffield Council on Bioethics.

Salvi, M. (2003) Conflict of interest in biomedical research: A view from Europe. *Science and Engineering Ethics* **9**(1), 101–108.

Scott, P.A., Välimäki, M., Leino-Kilpi, H., Dassen, T., Gasull, M., Lemonidou, C., et al. (2003a) Autonomy, privacy and informed consent 1: Concepts and definitions. *British Journal of Nursing* **12**(1), 43–47.

Scott, P.A., Välimäki, M., Leino-Kilpi, H., Dassen, T., Gasull, M., Lemonidou, C., et al. (2003b) Autonomy, privacy and informed consent 3: Elderly care perspective. *British Journal of Nursing* **12**(3), 158–168.

Shamoo, A. & Resnik, D. (2003) *Responsible conduct of research.* New York: Oxford University Press.

Spencer, C. (1997) A cuddle: A balance between beneficence and non-maleficence in the neonatal intensive care unit. *Journal of Neonatal Nursing* **3**(5), 29–33.

Stevens, P.E. & Pietsch, P.K. (2002) Informed consent and the history of inclusion of women in clinical research. *Health Care Women International* **23**(8), 809–819.

Stokamer, C.L. (2003) Pharmaceutical gift giving: Analysis of an ethical dilemma. *Journal of Nursing Administration* **33**(1), 48–51.

Touretzky, D.S. (1998) *Ethics and etiquette in scientific research.* Pittsburgh, PA: Carnegie Mellon University.

Veach, P.M., Bartels, D.M. & LeRoy, B.S. (2001) Ethical and professional challenges posed by patients with genetic concerns: A report of focus group discussions with genetic counselors, physicians, and nurses. *Journal of Genetic Counseling* **10**(2), 97–119.

Vogelsang, J. (1997) Plagiarism – an act of stealing. *Journal of Perianesthesia Nursing* **12**(6), 422–425.

World Health Organization (2000) *Operational guidelines for ethics committees that review biomedical research.* Geneva: World Health Organization.

Part 6
Research support

Chapter 18
Writing a research proposal

Karen H. Sousa & Marjolein M. Iversen

Introduction

When investigators want to study a phenomenon or issue, they prepare a formal research proposal and submit it to potential funders. The proposal is a detailed account of how the investigators will proceed and provides context for the study (Locke et al. 2000). A good proposal is very thorough – clear, concise, and complete – and presents enough detail that other researchers will be able to replicate the study. It also serves as a contract with the funder.

Writing a research proposal always entails far more work than the investigator anticipated. Even after many hours of preparation, there is no guarantee that potential funders will like it. Competition for research funding is tough – the number of applications is growing and only those of the highest quality are successful. Therefore, a proposal must make a strong argument that the study is critical and that the proposal's author is the right person to carry out the project (Boss & Eckert 2003).

This chapter offers guidance on writing a solid proposal and provides criteria for evaluating a draft so the author can improve it, thus making the proposal more persuasive.

Preparatory work

The first crucial step is to identify appropriate funders and learn about their priorities. Because these priorities change over time, the timing of a research proposal submission is key. Investigators also need to determine if their understanding of the phenomenon or issue to be studied matches the funder's understanding. The goal is to persuade the funder not only that the investigation is worthy, but also that the problem has been correctly defined (Locke et al. 2000).

Increasingly, funders are looking for innovative proposals that have an international focus and involve international cooperation. For example, all projects funded by the Research Council of Norway (2007) must have an international component, such as collaboration on publications.

Preparatory work includes carefully examining a funder's call for proposals and the deadline, establishing a writing schedule, and contacting consultants if their expertise will be necessary. Discussing a proposal with colleagues, mentors, and a funder's program officer can be helpful. In addition, what resources are available at the investigator's institution that may be useful? Grant-writing experts? Staff to help develop the study's budget? Library resources?

Applicants also should familiarize themselves with funding agencies' requirements for proposal format. For example, is there a limit on the number of pages? The proposal has to be reviewer friendly, with clearly labeled materials and appropriate figures and tables that enhance its readability. Overall, it must look professional.

Writing the proposal

The structure and style of a proposal depend largely on the funder's preferences, so the investigator should first decide which of the many different public and private funding sources he or she will target and then prepare a draft according to their guidelines. In any case, the proposal should tell a story. The elements of this story include:

- The phenomenon or issue and gap in knowledge;
- Why the study is important;
- The rationale for the study's approach;
- The country's broader research efforts or national priorities;
- The proposed study's objective and purpose;
- A basic description of the methodology and important potential outcomes;
- A description of related published research and why it is valuable; and
- Why the investigator thinks this story is exciting.

Using the funder's guidelines to evaluate the first draft may reveal weaknesses. When the applicant feels that all of the criteria have been met, the draft proposal is ready for review by one or more close colleagues or a mentor, who should receive a copy of the guidelines. Their critique can provide valuable insight.

Components of a proposal

Research proposals include sections on specific aims; background and significance, including the conceptual framework; preliminary studies; and research design and analysis.

Specific aims

This section puts the proposed study in context and identifies its purpose. The purpose, or overall goal, can be general or specific. A general purpose would be 'to describe the epidemiology of diabetic foot ulcers in a large Norwegian area.' A specific purpose would be 'to examine empirically the six dimensions of the Wilson and Cleary (1995) health-related quality of life (HRQOL) model in two populations living with chronic illnesses by assessing the unique contribution of each dimension and the relationships among the dimensions in estimating overall quality of life, and then to evaluate how the relationships change over time.'

The introductory paragraph must capture the reviewer's attention, like the first paragraph in a novel. It should address the question, 'So what?' Because this paragraph creates the first impression, it may be the most important one in the proposal.

Specific aims, research questions, or hypotheses identify the study variables and evolve from the statement of purpose (Burns & Grove 2005). The variables must be conceptually and operationally defined and linked to the conceptual framework and measurements. The aims outline the work to be carried out; everything in the proposal should relate to them somehow. They summarize the action ('to describe . . . ,' 'to compare . . . ,' 'to develop . . .') and specify what the study will investigate. An aim should have a measurable outcome – for example, 'to describe the prevalence of diabetic foot ulcers among people with diabetes' or 'to test the Wilson and Cleary (1995) HRQOL model to assess whether it fits the data of persons living with rheumatoid arthritis and AIDS.' A study's aims are more specific than its purpose.

The aims should not be too ambitious in scope; limiting them to three or four is best. The volume of work to be carried out should be realistic within the grant's timeframe. The aims may have to be refined many times before the research proposal is completed. Feedback from others will help shape aims so they better convey the investigator's message.

The hypothesis or research question should be closely connected to the specific aims. For example, 'What is the prevalence of self-reported diabetic foot ulcers among people with type 1 and type 2 diabetes in a population-based study in the period 2006–2008?'

Answers to the following questions will help applicants to assess their specific aims section:

- Is the research problem clearly presented?
- Is the research problem significant for nursing and does the section adequately address the significance?
- Is the proposal driven by strong, well-defined aims?
- Does the topic fit the funder's agenda?

The entire section should be limited to one page that can stand on its own.

Background and significance

The background and significance section summarizes the phenomenon or issue to be studied, as well as current knowledge and knowledge gaps; emphasizes the phenomenon's or issue's importance; explains why a new study is necessary; and relates the study topic to nursing practice or patient care. Background and significance need to be clearly linked to the specific aims. This section also may include key related theories and possible solutions.

The background need not be a comprehensive review of published studies, but references must be relevant. It should also explain why the proposed study population is appropriate for answering the research question, how the results will contribute to knowledge or better health, and, if possible, how the study would become a model for research in other areas. If the study is related to broader initiatives or other funded projects that the principal investigator or research team is working on, this should be mentioned.

A literature review helps establish the significance of a proposed study. The review summarizes and critiques the most important theoretical and empirical knowledge (Burns & Grove 2005). It may briefly cite only recent studies or more extensively describe and critique a number of recent and historically significant studies. In either case, it should demonstrate that the principal investigator has a command of both current knowledge and knowledge regarding the topic to be investigated. The major constructs or keywords in the specific aims can be used as sub-headings in the literature review to organize it.

Either before or after the review, the investigator should discuss the proposed study's conceptual framework. This theoretical discussion connects the variables within the context of existing knowledge and to the research plan. Investigators use it to link the research problem to relevant theories in nursing or related fields and to develop a hypothesis for their own findings (Talbot 1995). The theoretical concepts and relationships between them are often presented in a graphic.

Answers to the following questions will help applicants assess the background and significance section:

- Is this section reader-friendly?
- Is the literature review thorough yet concise?
- Does the section critically review current knowledge about the study topic?
- Does it reflect the investigator's thorough knowledge of the topic?
- Is the section well-organized and does it incorporate the key study variables?
- Do the specific aims and/or hypotheses flow naturally from the conceptual framework?

Preliminary studies

This section gives applicants an opportunity to persuade reviewers that they have the skills and experience necessary to carry out the study. It can include a description of research the principal investigator has previously carried out, preliminary data from current studies or data that support the main hypothesis and feasibility of the prospective study, and the investigator's dissertation, published work, or other relevant professional information. Experience using the proposed research method, and evidence of successful previous collaborations, are also worth mentioning. In addition, the section should discuss the merits of the research team.

Here is an example of an introductory paragraph in the preliminary studies section:

> Following graduation, Dr. Sousa obtained research funding to further her programme of research, which involves patient outcomes, primarily HRQOL. To enhance her knowledge of structural equation modeling (SEM), Dr. Sousa has completed post-doctorate SEM workshops, such as 'AMOS, A Structural Equation Modeling Tool for Teaching and Research and Structural Equation Modeling Using LISREL,' at the Spring Institute, the University of British Columbia. She has also attended classes at Arizona State University focusing on SEM, mixed models, and multi-level modeling. Her application of SEM as a statistical approach for data analysis is making a unique contribution to the understanding of HRQOL, its predictors, and how it changes over time. The following are examples of funded studies that are directly related to the aims of this proposal.

Questions for assessing the preliminary studies section include these:

- Is there ample pilot work to support the specific aims of the proposed study?
- Is there evidence that the principal investigator's previous work has prepared him or her for the study?
- If the principal investigator will work alone, does he or she have the necessary experience? If researchers will collaborate, is the team sufficiently strong?

Design and analysis

Reviewers will better understand a proposed project if this section begins with a brief outline of the study design. The section should be succinct yet include ample details that demonstrate why the investigator chose a particular methodology. The methodology will determine the number of sub-sections, which should be clearly identified. Possible headings in the section are 'Design and Setting,' 'Sample,' 'Data Collection and Measurements,' 'Data Analysis,' and 'Protection of Human Subjects.' If the study will be experimental and include an intervention, the investigator must discuss the intervention protocols and the rationale for each of them.

Design and setting

This sub-section clearly states the type of design ('a population-based, cross-sectional study,' 'a cross-sectional study using focus groups,' 'a randomized controlled intervention study') and the research setting briefly described ('the diabetes outpatient clinic at a University Medical Centre,' 'primary health care centers in California').

Sample

Reviewers expect a description of the sampling method and a concise justi-
fication for it. Increasingly, they also expect a power analysis, which, before the
research proposal is submitted, determines the appropriate sample size. Early
consideration of sample size is important because it may have a major impact
on how a study is organized – for example, whether the research can be conducted at one site or will require multiple sites, or whether particular outcome
measures are feasible.

This sub-section should also describe the study population, specifying who
will be eligible to participate based on certain criteria ('adults older than 20 who
reside in the study area,' 'individuals living with AIDS who were diagnosed after
2000'). Investigators planning population-based research need to explain how
their study will encompass the whole population and then justify this approach.
Case–control researchers must specify how they will select cases and controls,
and those planning a randomized controlled trial should describe the randomization procedure. Regardless of the type of design, the proposal needs to present a plan for dealing with subject attrition. It is also important to cite
extraneous variables that will have to be controlled according to inclusion and
exclusion criteria.

Data collection and measurement

For intervention studies, investigators should describe the intervention and
comparison groups, the main exposure(s) and/or outcome(s) to be assessed, how
the intervention will be administered, and how its impact will be measured –
with questionnaires, biological samples, or other tools. The use of particular
tools must be justified in terms of their reliability, validity, scoring, and level
of measurement. This information can be organized and presented in tables.
Investigators who conduct intervention or cohort studies need to explain how
they will follow up with patients.

This sub-section also explains the procedures for collecting data, including
where and when the information will be gathered; training research assistants;
maintaining quality control to ensure data integrity; and paying stipends.
Researchers who gained such experience from previous studies should reference
those studies. Copies of the interview questions, scales, physiologic instruments,
or other tools, and permissions to use copyrighted materials, appear in appendices.

Data analysis

The data analysis sub-section briefly describes the types of analyses that will
be performed and their level of measurement, and lists alternative methods if
problems arise. If the study will use a new analytical method, its relevance for
future research should be mentioned.

The sub-section is presented in a way that links each aim with the analysis
method. Here are two examples:

(1) *Aim*: Using the confirmatory approaches of SEM, evaluate the construct
validity of both the English- and Spanish-language versions of the Pediatric
Asthma Quality of Life Questionnaire (PAQLQ). Confirmatory factor

analysis, using the theoretical structure of the PAQLQ (Figure 1), will be done in both the English- and Spanish-language population groups.

(2) *Aim*: Assess preventive foot care practices among Norwegians with diabetes. The research questions are: (i) What is the regularity of preventive foot care among persons with diabetes in Norway? (ii) What demographic, lifestyle, and disease-related factors are associated with preventive foot care? To analyze the first question, descriptive statistics (mean, standard deviation, percentages) will be calculated for demographic, lifestyle, and disease-related variables, and variables related to health care setting, diabetes examination, and foot inspection. To analyze the second question, bivariate analysis and multiple logistic regression will be performed (Iversen et al. 2008).

The applicant should also explain how the data will be cleaned and analyzed, and how individual hypotheses will be tested.

The sub-section usually concludes with a discussion of the study's limitations and a plan for communicating the findings. Potential limitations include weaknesses in the design, sampling method, instruments, data collection procedures, and generalizability of the study findings (Burns & Grove 2005). Some funders want a list of papers that will be published, while others expect applicants to discuss dissemination alternatives, such as presentations at conferences. If the investigator is applying for PhD funding, the prospective funder may request a brief description of papers the study could generate, including background, research questions, data analysis, and the tentative title of each paper. One option is to cite journals whose audiences would be interested in the study's findings.

Questions for assessing the proposal's sub-sections include:

- Is the design appropriate for the specific aims?
- Does the proposal explain why the selected statistical analyses are suitable for the study's level of measurement?
- Is the sample size adequate for all of the proposed sub-analyses?
- Is it easy to follow exactly what is being proposed, how the objectives will be achieved, and by whom?
- Is consultants' role well-defined?

Protection of human subjects

International agreements include guidelines for protecting human research subjects. In the USA, federal policy governs all research involving humans and conducted or supported by any federal department or agency, or subject to federal regulation. Some universities require that investigators complete courses or modules in ethics before they send out research proposals. Scientists are obligated to protect the life, health, privacy, and dignity of study participants and to consider all relevant ethical issues (World Medical Association 2008).

Ethical issues vary depending on the study, but they arise in all research projects. Some studies elicit few ethical concerns, while others, especially those related to public health, may stir a great deal of controversy. To avoid harming study participants, investigators must carefully consider the ethical implications when they plan a study – for example, the fact that subjects in the control group will not receive a possibly beneficial treatment or the possibility that exploration of sensitive themes may cause psychologic distress. Researchers in the USA typically cite the institutional review board they have asked, or will ask, for permission to proceed. If multiple institutions collaborate on a study, each may have to grant approval.

In this sub-section, investigators describe how they will protect the rights of study subjects and minimize risks to them. In particular, the sub-section should include a statement citing confidentiality safeguards and explain that researchers will obtain informed consent from subjects. Other ethics-related topics to be addressed are the demographic characteristics of participants, the sources of data about individually identifiable participants, the recruitment plan, and a discussion of why risks are warranted (Polit & Beck 2008). If the sample will include children, mentally impaired persons, or other vulnerable individuals, the proposal needs to explain why their participation is essential and how their rights will be protected – for example, that prospective subjects will not be coerced to participate, that those who decline to participate will not face discrimination when they seek health care, and that prospective subjects will receive information about risks and benefits.

These questions help assess the sub-section:

- Is there sufficient detail explaining how subjects will be protected from unnecessary physical harm or psychologic distress?
- Does the proposal fully describe the risks and benefits?
- Does it address informed consent?

Budget

The budget is not part of the study protocol, but it is an essential part of the funding application. Funders often have their own application forms, which usually include one for the budget.

On this form, the applicant should list all tasks related to the study's objectives and estimate how much time each will require. The total amount of funding necessary for staff, the largest expense, is calculated based on how much time individual researchers will contribute and their salaries. Each budget item must be justified. Other potential costs are those for data collection, travel, consultants, financial incentives for study participants, office supplies, and developing and publishing the results. The budget should only include items that the funder, in its instructions, has specified it will cover; otherwise, the applicant risks annoying reviewers and losing a funding opportunity.

Questions for assessing the budget section include:

- Is the budget within the funder's limits?
- Has the applicant identified all potential costs and appropriately justified them?
- Is the amount of requested funds in line with the study design and personnel who will contribute?

Evaluation criteria

Researchers can evaluate their draft proposal using criteria related to the study's significance, approach, innovation, investigators, and environment (National Institutes of Health 2004).[1]

Significance

A proposal must make the case that the study will tackle an important and meaningful problem or question, and that the solution or answer is worth finding. Does previous research, personal experience, or a theory support the need for a new study? How will the scientific and/or clinical community benefit if the study achieves its stated aims?

Approach

Considerations regarding the study approach include the appropriateness of the conceptual framework, design, methods, and analysis. Is the methodology sound? Is it the right one to answer the research question? Principal investigators insert their study into a line of inquiry and a developing body of knowledge by devising a conceptual framework founded on current knowledge, by making hypotheses emerge from answered and unanswered questions, and by selecting research methods based on previous work (Locke et al. 2000). Does the proposal include a plan for observing events carefully and systematically? Does it thoroughly explain the study's implications? Is there acknowledgment and identification of potential problems and possible solutions?

Innovation

Applicants should demonstrate that their project is unique, fresh, and innovative – for example, that a successful nursing study will improve patient care. Does the proposal describe novel concepts, study approaches, or methods for assessing an issue or problem?

Investigators

Applicants must convince reviewers that members of the research team have adequate training and experience to conduct the study. The scope of a project – which will be broader in multisite, randomized controlled trials and narrower in descriptive research – determines how much training and experience are necessary. Does the principal investigator's previous research suggest that he or she understands the topic well enough to accomplish the study's aims?

Environment

Investigators must show that the infrastructure of the organization or site where the research is to take place will contribute to the probability of success. Infrastructure includes support staff, equipment, supplies, and arrangements for handling confidential information. Are qualified data collectors available? Do researchers have access to library materials and other documents they may need? Is there statistical support? Are mechanisms in place to track and monitor expenditures?

Finishing touches

Brief profiles of research team members add a finishing touch to the proposal; they give reviewers a better sense of who will be contributing. Another touch is making sure that terms in the proposal match those in the funder's guidelines, and including common, discipline-specific keywords.

Finally, while reviewers are supposed to evaluate research proposals thoroughly, many only read the abstract and look at the study's aims, due to time constraints. Because they may score the merit of proposals based on either a complete or cursory review, the abstract and study aims warrant special attention as the applicant drafts them. They should be clearly written and, on their own, accurately reflect the substance of the entire proposal.

Summary

Growing competition for research funding dictates that research proposals be clear, concise, and complete, as well as persuasive. This chapter described the steps applicants should take in preparing a sound proposal – from preparatory work to presenting comprehensive study information in a way that adheres to funders' guidelines. Key components of a proposal include specific aims, background and significance, preliminary studies, and design and analysis. Equally important is the estimated budget; expenses must be justified and not exceed a funder's limitations. Numerous criteria are available to help applicants assess their proposals before they submit them, increasing the likelihood of success.

Note

1   Other helpful resources are niaid.nih.gov/ncn/grants/charts/checklists.htm, and Polit and Beck (2008).

References

Boss, J.M. & Eckert, J.H. (2003) Academic scientists at work: I can't believe they didn't like it! Part II: grant proposals. ScienceCareers.org, December 12, 1–4.

Burns, N. & Grove, S.K. (2005) *The practice of nursing research: Conduct, critique, and utilization*, 5th Edn. Philadelphia: W.B. Saunders.

Iversen, M.M., Ostbye, T., Clipp, E., Midthjell, K., Uhlving, S., Graue, M., et al. (2008) The regularity of preventive foot care in persons with diabetes. Results from the Nord-Trøndelag Health Study. *Research in Nursing and Health* 31(3), 226–237.

Locke, L.F., Spirduso, W.W. & Silverman, S.J. (2000) *Proposals that work: A guide for planning dissertations and grant proposals*, 4th Edn. Thousand Oaks, CA: Sage Publications.

National Institutes of Health (NIH) (2004) *NIH announces updated criteria for evaluating research grant applications*. Bethesda, MD: National Institutes of Health.

Polit, D.F. & Beck, C.T. (2008) *Nursing research: Principals and methods*, 8th Edn. Philadelphia: Lippincott Williams & Wilkins.

Research Council of Norway (2007) *Main strategy of the Research Council*. Oslo: Research Council of Norway.

Talbot, L.A. (1995) *Principles and practice of nursing research*. St. Louis, MO: Mosby.

Wilson, I.B. & Cleary, P.D. (1995). Linking clinical variables with health-related quality of life: A conceptual model of patient outcomes. *J Am Med Assoc* 273, 59–65.

World Medical Association (2008) *World Medical Association Declaration of Helsinki, Amended*. Geneva: World Medical Association.

Chapter 19
Planning and managing a research project

Sarie Human

Introduction

Successful research depends largely on clearly understanding a study's purpose and conducting the study in a scientifically rigorous way. It also depends on good planning and management, which are very important for maintaining the focus and integrity of a project and for dealing with differences in contributors' interpretations, expectations, and personal agendas.

Collaborators bring a wealth of knowledge and skills – as well as different experience and professional and cultural backgrounds – to a study. No less important are the research assistants, field workers, data coders, statisticians, editors, critical reviewers, community gatekeepers, and others who provide support. Because collaborations entail recruiting and overseeing numerous players, many of whom may work at multiple sites, they pose significant planning and management challenges. They also raise potentially thorny issues regarding the responsibilities and rights of contributors, ownership of data, communication among team members, and scientific and ethical rigor.

This chapter focuses on how to plan and manage collaborative research to maximize its efficiency and effectiveness, and reviews issues the nurse scientist may encounter as a member of the research team.

Planning

Planning is about structure, order, and effective management of research, including breaking a project into smaller and more manageable units, goals, stepping stones, and timeframes. Collaborators initially meet to clarify and agree on a number of issues, including roles and responsibilities, formulation of the research question, goals, methodology, the meaning and interpretation of operational definitions, sampling, research processes, communication strategies, ethical and financial concerns, record-keeping, follow-up meetings, and timelines. Planning also addresses field worker training, timely printing and distribution of instruments, focus group logistics, interpretation of data, peer review, quality assurance and data validation, travel and subsistence allowances, and feedback from all stakeholders when the project ends. In addition, investigators need to consider publication-related issues. Whose names will appear as authors on the final report? Should the researchers publish one article or a series of articles? Where should the results be published (a decision that might best wait until the findings emerge)?

Committees subsequently are assigned certain tasks. Among them are reviewing the literature, designing protocols, developing measurement tools, preparing a budget and necessary documents, identifying and seeking permission from gate-keepers who must authorize research, and assembling training materials.

The budget

Planning the budget can be difficult, as many variables that may not be entirely clear at the time of planning warrant consideration. Aside from individual expenses, such variables include inflation; the length of the study; the total number of contributors, support staff, and study subjects; the number and nature of team meetings; printing needs; and courier services versus postage, especially if the local postal system is not reliable. The advice of experienced researchers is useful in compiling a feasible, affordable, and appropriate budget.

The budget should include the estimated cost of these items:

- Remuneration for researchers and support staff. The amount may be based on formulas that account for the expertise of participants, their level of participation and the time they contribute, their salaries, and what they will deliver. Team members need to agree on the remuneration formula, which must be specified in formal agreements. Payment is typically linked to deliverables and made in three or four installments or as a lump sum at the end of the project.
- Remuneration for study subjects. In many countries, especially in the developing world, researchers offer incentives, such as shopping vouchers for food

or other personal necessities, rather than money. The budget should also include participants' travel, food, and accommodation expenses. Investigators must carefully consider this issue when planning the budget because the type of remuneration may have scientific and ethical implications.

- Temporary administrative support, an important component of successful research. Administrative staff manage the printing and distribution of materials; make travel arrangements; arrange for venues, transportation, accommodations, and catering; keep financial records; and organize meetings and take minutes.
- Equipment, including laptop computers, printers, telephones, office space, and stationery.
- Postage, printing, and other communication needs.
- Meetings, training, quality control and data validation, statistical support, and data entry and analysis.

The primary investigator's role

Although the primary investigator (PI) directs, manages, and monitors a study, and therefore carries the ultimate responsibility, everyone who collaborates or provides support is accountable for meeting professional standards, including standards for scientific and ethical rigor.

Ethical reviews

Obtaining permission for research from institutional reviews boards and community gatekeepers is primarily the PI's responsibility. In multiple-site studies, the PI may delegate responsibility for obtaining institutional or health authority permission to collaborators who will oversee the research at those sites or in particular geographic areas.

Direction and guidance

Before research begins, all collaborators and support staff must agree on the study's purpose, methodology, expectations, interpretations, strategies, course of action, and operational processes. The PI should give them direction and guidance, as well as clarification and support, throughout the project and at regular, planned intervals. He or she may also need to help resolve problems and, when necessary, discipline contributors or support staff.

Control and monitoring

These critical PI tasks include making sure that the project adheres to timelines, verifying data accuracy and validity, managing data entry and analysis, monitoring record-keeping, providing opportunities for feedback, and scrutinizing the commitment and ethical rigor of research assistants. In addition, the PI must coordinate peer review and other critiques, quality assurance, and report writing and editing. He or she also is responsible for controlling and monitoring funds to ensure they are spent properly.

Communication

PIs have a 'finger on the pulse' of research and serve as a kind of communication hub. They maintain open communications among team members and keep them informed and updated about progress, challenges, deadlines, findings, problems in the field, solutions to those problems, and more. Their communications help clarify concepts and procedures, foster momentum and enthusiasm, and are supportive of team members.

Good communication among all players – whether in face-to-face meetings, e-mail, conversations, text messages via cell phone, video conferences, or Internet-based chat rooms or discussion forums – is at the foundation of collaboration. This requires attention to regular communications, good people skills, acknowledgment of individual contributions, maintaining the research focus, and monitoring feasibility. For example, face-to-face meetings every month may not be feasible; perhaps bi-monthly meetings with teleconferences in between would be better. Perhaps some procedures, materials, or services are not affordable, given the project's budget. Other issues in which communication may have a key role include study subjects' acceptance of the research and the ethical behavior of collaborators. During a project, staff training, the availability of facilities and equipment, and many other issues can arise, all of which require that participants confer with each other.

Self-discipline and a commitment by all team members to communicate routinely and clearly, and to adhere to procedures and timelines, are essential elements of effective communication. There need to be planned opportunities for them to communicate freely and provide feedback on the study's progress, challenges, successes, and strategies.

Quality assurance

High-quality research often requires the knowledge and expertise of support personnel, such as statisticians, editors, and critical reviewers. The PI must put the necessary controls in place to maintain quality. This responsibility includes budgeting time for quality assurance tasks – everything from thorough statistical analysis to critical reviews of the findings.

Mentorship

All research projects involve learning from others. PIs have an important role in this regard by organizing their study in a way that promotes mentorship – pairing a less-experienced or less-skilled member of the research team with a more seasoned investigator or field worker. PIs can also indirectly promote these educational relationships by creating learning opportunities, monitoring the progress of mentorships, offering direction and advice, supporting and listening to mentees, helping to solve problems, and conducting informative and open discussions.

For mentorships to thrive, team members must be committed to sharing information, knowledge, and skills, and to putting the study's purpose and goals ahead of personal agendas and expectations.

Assembling and managing a team

Research that relies on a variety of collaborators is both beneficial and challenging. To maximize the benefits and minimize the challenges, investigators must take numerous factors into account when assembling and managing a team.

Recruitment

The first step in recruitment is to identify assistance needs and then find the right people to meet them. Recruiting collaborators and support staff involves the following considerations:

- How important are specific types of expert knowledge and skills?
- Is adequate representation of cultural groups, geographic locations, or other factors a necessity?
- What, if any, interest groups related to the study population will be involved? Community gatekeepers? Authorities whose permission to conduct the research may be necessary? Groups to provide feedback on the findings?
- Should the study include learning opportunities for novice researchers and/or students?
- Must the researchers find institutions or organizations willing to fund or sponsor their study?

Recruitment depends on the availability of certain expertise, knowledge, cultural views, and professional and life experiences. A diversity of contributors can make it difficult to balance and harmonize different views, expectations, and opinions, but if conflicts are managed proactively and sensitively, diversity always produces better research results.

A lack of commitment to the research goals, and personality clashes or professional jealousy, are detrimental. Experience has shown that it is better to lose or replace troublesome collaborators than retain their valuable expertise. A study's objectives must always be a greater priority than individual views, agendas, and perceptions.

Good teamwork requires a clear understanding of individual roles and responsibilities, which need to be spelled out in formal agreements before research begins.

Roles and responsibilities

Formal agreements with collaborators and support staff include details about roles and responsibilities, expectations, proper procedures, remuneration, and a remediation process if a team member does not deliver work on time or if the team agrees that, in the project's best interest, the individual should no longer participate.

The PI needs to facilitate, rather than dictate, the finalization of these issues. Among the goals of collaborative research are to arrive at the best possible decisions based on broad input and to give all participants an opportunity to buy into and own the project. When a conflict or disagreement arises, first the PI and then the team needs to address it openly and as sensitively and quickly as possible. Effective teams flourish in a transparent and trusting research environment.

Conflicts of interest

Researchers should identify and declare conflicts of interest, and discuss them with team members, to prevent bias and damage to a study's credibility. Such conflicts may be related to funding, sampling, questions for study subjects, data collection or analysis, interpretation of findings, or recommendations. They may have to be addressed in formal agreements before research begins – if, for example, a team member has a financial interest in the shop where computers for the study will be purchased.

The type of conflict of interest and its potential impact on a study will guide the decision about whether the individual should withdraw from the project or only certain aspects of it. When a conflict is known and the individual does not withdraw, careful monitoring and quality control are necessary.

Training

Even though many team members may have vast experience in their particular field, every research project is unique and entails some degree of learning and training. All participants must have the knowledge and skills necessary to complete their assigned tasks. This is especially true for inexperienced field workers who will conduct interviews or collect other types of data, as a study's validity, reliability, and ethical integrity will largely depend on their skills. The study plan should address field worker training, if training is necessary, and strategies for assessing the completeness and accuracy of the data they gather. All members of the research team must be aware of and agree to such strategies, with the aim of facilitating a positive learning environment instead of an authoritative or punitive one.

Training can empower people and transfer knowledge and research skills that will benefit them during and after a project.

Data ownership

Ownership of data is often a contentious issue that collaborative researchers and participating entities need to discuss and address in formal agreements. Among the many questions it raises are the following:

- Do the data, and therefore the findings, belong to the entity that commissioned the study, to the study sponsor, to the researcher, or to a government health authority? Who owns the copyright?
- What rights do participating academic institutions have in terms of accessing and using the data?
- Who should have access to the data? Only the PI? The PI and collaborators? The study participants?
- Who should receive authorship credit?
- Who is entitled to publish what, and where?

- How will the publication process work?
- Who is responsible for getting the final report published?
- Who should give permission for publication?
- What are contributors' rights and responsibilities regarding published results?
- Who is entitled to benefit financially or in any other way from publication?
- When will data ownership expire, thus enabling others to use the information for their own purposes?

An ethical issue that may arise is pressure from a stakeholder in the study to show that the findings prove a theory or validate a position the stakeholder embraces. If the results do not meet such expectations, the stakeholder might try to prohibit publication in the scientific or public domain.

The following factors typically influence decisions about data ownership:

- A contentious or sensitive research topic, such that publication will have negative implications for one or more stakeholders;
- An official study sponsor that claims ultimate control over the data and report;
- Researchers' expectations, rights, and responsibilities;
- The legal implications if findings are published, especially when research involves children or other vulnerable groups;
- A study seeks to influence policy, advocate for a vulnerable group, or explore new trends; and
- The manner of results reporting and dissemination, including the journal in which they will appear and the timing of publication.

Informed consent

Informed consent, a basic ethical issue, entails multiple permissions – from the entity or community gatekeeper that has authority over the study population and from all study subjects. The latter must clearly understand their rights and the study's implications, and have complete freedom to agree or decline to participate.

Although the PI is primarily responsible for informed consent, field workers are obligated to ensure that all study participants are fully aware of the research purpose, the type of information they will be asked to provide, the data collection method, how the information will be used, confidentiality safeguards, and their right to withdraw at any time. Data collectors should address participants' expectations that may arise as a result of questions asked. For example, if a researcher asks children with HIV/AIDS what they ate the previous day, it could create an expectation that the researcher will provide food.

If information that study subjects will provide is very sensitive or if experiences they report might evoke strong emotions or psychologic reactions, investigators should make counselors and/or support structures available and tell participants about the availability of such. Collaborators need to address this issue in the study planning stage. HIV/AIDS, rape, child abuse, traumatic loss of family members or friends, life-threatening conditions that led to disfiguring surgery, and other topics can be very troubling for participants.

Most researchers obtain informed consent in writing so they have a record, although fingerprints are acceptable when study subjects are illiterate. When participants are minors, mentally disabled, or vulnerable in some other way, investigators must adhere to laws about obtaining informed consent from parents and/or guardians, and thoroughly discuss the related ethical issues. Thorough discussion is also necessary, along with agreement among all stakeholders, when participants are willing to give only oral consent because of the sensitivity of the research topic. In these cases, investigators must carefully consider the type of data they will need, and the appropriateness, ethical integrity, and implications of oral consent.

Interdisciplinary collaboration

Interdisciplinary collaboration is advantageous because it pools knowledge, skills, and perspectives from various disciplines. It also may enhance the usability and acceptability of findings over a broader field and across disciplines.

The entire research team must maintain and monitor a balance among the research focus, professional bias, and interdisciplinary competition. One profession should not unnecessarily dominate, which can occur if a collaborator is more experienced or more knowledgeable about the study topic than others, or if he or she has a dominating personality.

Clearly specified roles, regular and effective communication, and good quality control are important building blocks of successful interdisciplinary collaborations.

Challenges in nursing research

Independent nurse investigators

In many countries, because of historical and other factors, nurses and nursing do not have the status of professions in the natural sciences, such as medicine. Often, nurses collect data as part of their day-to-day activities without official recognition of their role as collaborators. Or they may not have the confidence, time, skills, or research orientation to initiate and complete studies independently.

Nursing includes aspects of both the social and natural sciences, which some natural scientists cite as a reason to disregard it as a scientific profession. Therefore, nursing curricula must have sound scientific and analytic underpinnings, and research mindedness and skills must be cultivated at all levels of nursing practice.

A second challenge for independent nurse researchers in numerous countries is that their work often does not result in scientifically accredited or peer-reviewed publication, perhaps because they do not pursue publication or their studies are viewed as too narrowly focused. They can enhance the relevance of their work, and its impact on nursing science and nursing practice, by collaborating with other health professionals.

Thirdly, many nurses have difficulty obtaining research funding. Medical investigators and those who conduct experimental studies, such as clinical trials, typically receive funding preference over investigators who conduct qualitative research.

Finally, many national and international scientific journals are biased against nursing research. Journals typically pay greater attention to medicine and other fields, especially in countries where pure nursing research is not deemed to be 'scientific.' Nurse scientists can overcome such challenges by forming research groups and networks, which have more impact than individual investigators and extend the profession's collective research capacity.

Nurse collaborators

Nurses often are collaborative team members in research projects because of their sheer number and availability in clinical settings. They may be their own worst enemies by agreeing to collect data or serve as field workers without receiving any recognition in published articles or having opportunities to contribute at a meaningful scientific level. Nurses should know their rights as co-researchers and co-authors. They deserve recognition as scientists.

To participate in collaborative and interdisciplinary studies as equal and recognized team members, nurses must continuously develop and update their scientific knowledge and research skills. Recognition is not a right; it must be earned through credibility and high-quality contributions to research.

Nurses often are in a unique position among members of a research team because, in addition to providing scientific input, they advocate for patients, vulnerable groups, and communities.

Maintaining a nursing focus

As part of a research team, nurse scientists must be vigilant for influences that can hijack a study's nursing focus, such as competing research priorities, funding availability, sponsors' expectations, and domination by other disciplines. They must also help keep nursing issues on national, regional, and local research agendas.

Summary

In collaborative research, investigators tap a variety of expertise and other resources. This model brings a valuable diversity of professional knowledge and experience to research projects, but it also presents many challenges, which can be overcome through careful planning and management. A key planning task is preparing an estimated budget that accounts for all anticipated expenses.

The principal investigator has a lead role in managing research. He or she is responsible for ethical behavior, providing direction and guidance, controlling and monitoring the entire process to ensure that a study adheres to timelines and is scientifically rigorous, facilitating communication, maintaining quality, and fostering mentorship. Assembling and managing a research team includes recruiting the right people, assigning clear roles and responsibilities, addressing conflicts of interest, and training team members. Among the critical issues that collaborators must not overlook are data ownership and informed consent.

Nurse scientists face a number of unique obstacles – from bias against nursing research in many countries to funding-related hurdles. However, by keeping their knowledge and research skills current, and joining groups or networks that bolster the profession's research capacity, nurses can make meaningful contributions to scientific collaborations.

Further reading

Allen, D. & Lyne, P. (2006) *The reality of nursing research: Politics, practices, and processes.* London: Routledge.

Baier, D., Decker, R. & Schmidt-Thieme, L. (Eds) (2005) *Data analysis and decision support.* New York: Springer-Verlag.

Bak, N. (2004) *Completing your thesis; A practical guide.* Pretoria: Van Schaik Publishers.

Brink, H. (2006) *Fundamentals of research methodology for health care professionals,* 2nd Edn. Cape Town: Juta and Company.

Dlugacz, Y.D. (2006) *Measuring health care.* San Francisco: Jossey-Bass.

Fitzpatrick, J. & Montgomery, K.S. (2004) *Internet for nursing research: A guide to strategies, skills and resources.* New York: Springer Publishing.

Henning, E., Van Rensburg, W. & Smit, B. (2004) *Finding your way in qualitative research.* Pretoria: Van Schaik Publishers.

Koshy, V. (2005) *Action Research for improving practice: A practical guide.* London: Paul Chapman Publishing.

Mouton, J. (2001) *How to succeed in your master's and doctoral studies: A South African guide and resource book.* Pretoria: Van Schaik Publishers.

Richards, L. (2005) *Handling qualitative data: A practical guide.* London: Sage Publications.

Willis, J.W. (2007) *Foundations of quality research: Interpretive and critical approaches.* London: Sage Publications.

Chapter 20
Presenting and publishing research findings

Leana R. Uys

Introduction

A research proposal implies that a study will contribute to knowledge and influence peoples' lives. However, this can happen only if the results are presented and/or published, which means research is not completed until investigators have taken this final step. Other researchers, policy-makers, and the public may question the ethical behavior of an investigator who fails to make findings accessible to them.

There are many reasons why researchers do not disseminate or publish study findings. The most common one is that the researchers merely seek a higher degree or tenure. In many developing countries, unpublished studies may be the only kind that nurses pursue as their profession grows and matures over many years. Not publishing results seems like a significant waste of time and effort, even though the studies may have limitations. Among the reasons researchers cite for not publishing are a preoccupation with teaching or work on a new project, disappointing study results, poor presentation skills, or ignorance about article preparation. Although these may be legitimate barriers, all researchers should commit to the dissemination of findings and develop the necessary skills.

Audiences for research findings

It is important to think carefully about how to share findings. This involves targeting one or more of four audiences: professional colleagues, other investigators with an agenda or project that may be influenced by the results, policy-makers and administrators, and the community.

Because many nurses do not read the scientific literature, investigators may have to disseminate their findings to professional colleagues in other ways. These include giving talks at local professional meetings, participating in continuing education, or writing articles for professional publications rather than scientific journals that have a research focus. Such articles provide few details about a study; instead, they summarize the results and their overall implications for nursing practice.

The second type of audience, other researchers, may be interested in more than a study's findings, such as the theoretical framework, methodology, definitions, measurement tools, sample size, access to study participants, or data analysis technique. Investigators can reach this group by speaking at research conferences, presenting posters, or publishing in journals.

If findings have policy implications, often the best way to get research findings implemented is to present them to the third type of audience – policy-makers and administrators – perhaps in the form of a written brief sent by mail. At the local level, policy-makers may be chief nurses or health officials, many of whom do not read research journals. Nationally or internationally, they may include health service planners, politicians, managers of aid agencies, and nurse leaders in professional organizations or regulatory bodies.

The fourth audience, the community at large, is especially important if the research was community-based. This group owns the information that study participants gave to data collectors. The community might need the findings to lobby for changes in health care delivery or its members may change their health behavior based on the findings. In addition, dissemination teaches a community about the value of research, such that the community may be more inclined to support future projects. Presentation of results can take place at a community meeting or through media such as local newspapers or radio stations. The sampling method is always of great interest to the audience, often raising questions such as, 'Why did you talk to these particular people?' or 'Are your respondents really representative of the whole community?' It is important to present the results in enough detail so everyone understands them and to offer guidance on what the community can do about the research problem. The goal is to encourage appropriate action, not induce a feeling of powerlessness and anxiety.

Forms of presentation

Posters

A poster consists of pages mounted in a hall during a conference that describe the study, usually augmented by printed handouts and informal discussions between the author and viewers (Miller 2007). They enable maximum interaction between the presenter and audience, are an excellent alternative for researchers who lack formal presentation skills, and, at highly popular conferences, are more likely than formal presentations to be accepted.

Posters should address the interests of as many conference attendees as possible, who may be quite diverse and include scientists, educators, policy-makers, and practitioners. A good poster is simple, clear, and has relevant take-home messages. Because viewers stand and read posters in a bustling, distractive environment, the presentation must grab and hold their attention and be easy to read.

Among the essential elements of poster design are the following:

- It should focus on two or three main points, as one poster cannot describe a large project comprehensively.
- Depending on permissible size, the poster will have one to three columns of text. In a three-column presentation, the central column is usually twice the size of the other two.
- The title, authors' names, and affiliations appear at top center in a font of at least 40 points. Including e-mail addresses here is useful because handouts with this information may run out.
- Headings follow the IMRAD format – introduction, materials and methods, results, additions, and discussion. The introduction, materials/methods, and an abstract go in the first column, the results in the second column, and the discussion and acknowledgments in the third. References are not necessary.
- Clear, simple, titled figures are used to convey numeric data because they are easier and quicker to read than tables or narrative. Beneath each figure should be a few sentences describing the pattern it illustrates, including information about the magnitude and direction of the association between variables.
- Not all viewers have advanced statistical knowledge. If it is necessary to present statistics, 'keep the focus on your results, not the arithmetic needed to conduct inferential statistical tests' (Miller 2007, p. 315). One or two sentences that explain in simple terms what the investigator tried to establish through testing makes the results accessible to all.

A handout enables interested persons to take a copy of the poster with them. It can be a printed version of a PowerPoint slide or a single-page copy of the abstract and a few key figures. Providing a more comprehensive report or article reprint is expensive and saddles the viewer with a ream of paper to carry home. Exchanging business cards and e-mail addresses may be a better option.

Publication in professional journals

Getting published is essential for researchers who seek an academic career. In some professional circles, the number of published articles is of prime importance; in others, both the number and quality are important. In either case, the choice of publications tells potential employers something about the investigator, which is one reason to choose journals carefully. The following factors warrant consideration:

- It is best to avoid journals with a very small or local circulation that are not indexed in PubMed,[1] an international, open-access archive of health publications, or another major archive. The importance of a journal to its field is expressed in terms of an objective measure called the impact factor (IF), based on the frequency with which an average article in the journal has been cited by other researchers in a specified time period. The IF is usually cited on the home page of a journal's website; if not, one can e-mail the editor and ask for it. A journal that does not provide IFs probably has little international impact.
- Peer-reviewed journals have more credibility because critiques by experts before publication often improve articles significantly. Professionally, it is not advantageous for researchers to publish in obscure, non-peer-reviewed journals.

- Journals generally focus on a certain field, some more broadly than others. The more specialized the study, the more specialized the targeted journal should be. This enables the investigator to network with other researchers working in the same field and possibly collaborate with them in the future. Reading several issues of a publication may be the best way to determine if it is appropriate for a proposed article.

Journal websites are an important resource. They usually provide author guidelines that enable investigators to determine if a publication meets their particular needs. Certain journals publish lengthy clinical studies, others just brief reports. Some websites also have extensive guidelines regarding the proper format of submissions.

Adhering to a standard article format enables the researcher to present a maximum amount of information organized in an efficient way and makes it easier for readers to find the information they are seeking. The IMRAD format, discussed earlier regarding posters, also applies to many journal articles. The format is inappropriate for specific types of studies, such as historical research. Some authors customize IMRAD by adding their own components.

Essential elements that precede the IMRAD section of an article are:

- *Title*: should describe the content accurately and clearly so readers can decide if they want to read the article. Some journals prefer that the title be in the form of a question the article answers, while others prefer a title that summarizes the answer. Authors should avoid abbreviations, jargon, cute titles, and unnecessary words such as 'study of' (Day 2001).
- *Keywords*: not only accurately describe the article's thrust, but also enable someone to find related documents using an online search engine such as on PubMed. One way to choose keywords is to carry out a few searches in the relevant research field using different terms to see which yield the best results.
- *Authors*: 'The list of authors should accurately reflect who did the work' (Blackwell Publishing). Three criteria for citing authors are: '(1) substantial contributions to the conception, design, or acquisition of data or analysis and interpretation of data; (2) drafting the article or revising it critically for important intellectual content; and (3) final approval of the version to be published' (International Committee of Medical Journal Editors 2008, p. 3).
- *Abstract*: reflects the whole report in summarized form. Structured abstracts are better than unstructured ones because they make it easier for others who search the literature to identify relevant articles. This also facilitates literature reviews because, for some published articles, only abstracts are available (Nakayama et al. 2005). The IMRAD format is suitable for abstracts, although, for original articles, Guimaraes (2006) suggests a more extensive format comprising up to nine headings: objective, design, setting, patients or participants, interventions, main outcome measures, results, limitations, and conclusions. The headings for review articles are purpose, studies selected for review, data sources, data extraction, and results. Abstracts should not include references, figures, tables, or any information not in the article.

The IMRAD section begins with the introduction, which answers these questions: What is the problem? Why is it important? The introduction describes the problem in general terms, then presents current knowledge about it and the knowledge gaps. This provides context for the study. Importance has to do with the scope of the problem, the severity of its impact, conflicts between current solutions or theories, or other major implications. Finally, the introduction tells readers what the investigators examined and briefly describes the research questions and overall study design. The link between the problem and the study's focus must be clear.

The next topic, materials and methods, covers the research design, study population, sampling method and process, and instruments. It answers these questions: How did the investigators study the problem? What specific steps did they take? What tools did they use? The text should be sufficiently thorough that others could replicate the study or evaluate the validity and applicability of the results based on this information. Details are important – for example, the species and strain in an animal study, or the brand and year of software the investigators used. The order of information here corresponds to the study process. This is also where the author describes the study's ethical safeguards.

There are different ways to present the results. If investigators posed a number of research questions, they can answer each of them with the relevant findings. If there was only one research question, they typically describe the results in order of importance, without any interpretation.

In the IMRAD format, additions means tables and figures. The author should use only those that summarize and clarify complex data. Tables do not include data that can easily be described in one or two sentences. References in the narrative to data in the tables must not simply repeat the data.

Finally, the discussion addresses these questions: What do the results mean? What are their implications? What limitations did the study have? Day (2001) suggests that authors move from the specific to the general by summarizing the most important finding first and comparing it with existing knowledge in the literature, then address theory and, lastly, the implications for nursing practice, education (of health professionals, the general public, or other constituencies), and policy. The text should include a plausible explanation for both the expected and unexpected findings, and what the implications are for other theories. Do the results support or contradict those theories? Do the results raise new theoretical questions, and if so, what are they?

Acknowledgments appear after the IMRAD section. Authors are ethically obliged to disclose all sources of funding for the research and publication of results, even when they write related editorials or letters to the editor.

Publication in mass media

When writing for a wider audience than scientists, the author must make a greater effort to engage readers because they may not see how the topic relates to them. There are two major approaches: telling a story, or narrative journalism, and posing a problem.

Narrative journalism not only conveys information, but also enables the reader to 'experience' events through story-telling (Quinterno 2009). The author relays an individual's, family's, or community's experience in a highly personal and emotive way which includes many details and uses text boxes, tables, and/or graphs containing more scientific information to augment the storyline.

Readers are more likely to read to the end because the story stirs their emotions and feeds their minds, creating a powerful influence on behavior. Compared to facts alone, readers remember a story better and it affects their decisions for a longer period of time.

In the second approach, the author poses a problem that readers themselves may be experiencing and then presents information, based on the research findings, that will help them understand and possibly overcome it. This technique can link research to the everyday work world of practicing nurses or the daily experience of community members.

Articles for publication in mass media begin with a catchy, but also accurate and descriptive, title. The introduction sets the scene, explains the problem, presents characters, and describes action that unfolds over time from the perspective of the storyteller, who engages readers emotionally and then imparts information that will lead them to a point, realization, or destination (Kramer 2005). The article sketches the problem in a way that rings true to readers. Reporting on conversations or the author's own nursing experiences, supplemented with quotes and photographs, are helpful for this purpose.

The body of the article describes the research findings as a way to better understand or solve the problem. It does not discuss the research methodology; readers can learn more about that and other scientific details by referring to the original journal article.

The conclusion summarizes an easily remembered and useful take-home message.

Oral presentations

Investigators orally present their findings in various ways – by reading a paper at a conference, conducting a seminar with co-researchers, hosting a workshop to promote implementation of the findings, or speaking to the community where the study took place. The goals, structure, level of reported detail, and communication technology depend on the type of presentation.

For an oral presentation at a conference, the paper should adhere to the IMRAD format, with a summary slide for each component. Essential considerations in all oral presentations include the following:

- The presentation should not cover too much territory. It must summarize the content within the allotted time without requiring a quick delivery. The presenter can gauge the length by practicing in advance.
- The speaker should use audiovisual aids, such as PowerPoint slides, to keep the audience's attention and convey complex data.
- The full text of the presentation should be printed in a large font, with highlights in bold type, so the presenter can easily read it. Notations in the text indicate when the next slide is to appear. Highlights alone or a PowerPoint printout may be enough for experienced speakers.
- The speaker should be prepared for questions, as questions and answers are as important as the formal presentation. Colleagues can help by posing possible questions beforehand. At the podium, the presenter may repeat a question from the audience in his or her own words if its meaning is not entirely clear.

The appropriate speed for showing slides or overhead transparencies is about one per minute. It is better to use fewer slides if some of them have tables or charts, given that this kind of information takes more time to absorb. Slides must be in at least an 18-point font so the audience can read them. A printed hand-out of the slides enables audience members to review the information later.

In community-based and action research, the findings belong to the community as well as the investigator, who therefore must share the results publicly. At community gatherings, informal talks supplemented with handouts containing a few important tables or graphs are best. (Slides or overhead transparencies may not even be feasible.) Such talks focus on the study's purpose, how the researchers selected study participants, and the results and implications for the community. The talk should not focus only on the problem; it must also offer advice about how to address the problem, especially when research highlights a need to change a behavior, service, or policy. It may be appropriate to tell community groups about such needs so they can be informed consumers and take responsibility for their own health and health care.

Press releases

The press release is a form of persuasive communication written in a strict, journalistic style. It conveys the essential message of a published article in the most targeted manner possible. It also tries to 'sell' something without being overtly promotional (Hansen 2009). A press release is successful only if journalists who receive it think it is useful, interesting, and accurate.

Smart scientists sell their product (research results) to the public, decision-makers, and policy-makers through the mass media. By doing so, they bring news-worthy scientific work they and their institution are doing to the attention of community leaders, funding agencies, or other stakeholders, enhancing both the scientist's and the institution's reputations. Policy-makers are more likely to read a press release than a published article.

A press release is usually issued on the day the article is published. This draws attention to the article, thus promoting its content, the author(s), and the journal to a wide audience without infringing on the journal's exclusive copyright. Depending on a study's focus, the article may initiate a debate in the mass media, which seldom happens if journalists must learn about it on their own, without a press release.

Researchers who live in a multilingual country should consider making a press release available in more than one language. This is especially important if the investigator wants to inform communities in which the dominant language is not widely spoken. In addition, multilingual press releases greatly increase the chance of reaching those communities via journalists and editors.

In the case of international research, a press release is typically issued on the same day in all countries involved in the study, even if media interest is likely to vary.

The following guidelines will help authors prepare effective press releases (Stoller 2009):

- The focus should be clear.
- Releases are written on official letterhead in block style, without paragraph indentations. 'For immediate release' and the contact's name and phone number appear at the top.

- The headline, which highlights the most important, amazing, or impressive fact in the press release, must be short and snappy to grab journalists' attention and prompt them to read further. A longer sub-heading fleshes out the headline.
- The first line begins with the dateline (city and state).
- All of the essential information goes in the opening paragraph, with the news first and then the names of those who announced it. The writer should avoid excessive adjectives, flowery language, and hyperbole, and never use the pronoun 'I'.
- The second paragraph answers the who, what, why, where, and when questions. It often includes a quote to personalize the release.
- The body of the release comprises informative details that will spark more curiosity.
- The writing should be concise, factual, and as objective as possible. Shorter rather than longer is best – one page, ideally. The text is double-spaced and in one font, with page numbers. The writer must not embellish facts or make claims that cannot be substantiated.
- The last paragraph summarizes the release and tells readers who to contact and how for more information.
- The release concludes with '###' or '-30-,' a journalistic practice that indicates this is the end.
- Releases must be correct and accurate – no misspellings, grammatical mistakes, factual errors, or misquotes. Name spellings and titles should be double-checked for accuracy.
- Sending a release to familiar journalists or those whose beat matches the article topic, such as health, increases the likelihood it will generate interest.
- A follow-up phone call ensures that contacts received the press release.

Policy briefs

A policy brief is a document outlining the rationale for recommending a particular alternative or course of action in a current policy debate (Young & Quinn 2004). If a study has clear policy implications, the researcher might want to bring the results and implications to the attention of the appropriate authorities or decision-makers. Sometimes a brief is prepared by a lobbying group that advocates a specific policy; in other cases, a decision-maker requests one.

Policy briefs are a marketing tool. As such, they should be aimed at selling a specific policy to targeted decision-makers. If a decision-maker discusses or helps develop a brief, there must be adequate objective evidence to support it.

A good policy brief has the following characteristics:

- Focuses on only one problem or issue.
- Written in a professional, rather than a scientific, style. The brief should summarize a study's findings as evidence for the proposed policy, not describe the study's methodology or analytical procedures.
- Evidence-based and uses neutral, non-emotive language. It tries to persuade policy-makers with a rational and systematic argument rather than exhort, castigate, or shame them.

- Is precisely what it claims to be – brief, typically less than eight pages or 3000 words – to accommodate busy people who have little spare time. The font and lay-out should make the document an easy read.
- Written clearly and simply. One way to promote understanding is to use headings in the form of questions.

Developing a policy brief begins with a careful assessment of mainstream opinion in the literature – the pro and con arguments. This helps the author decide what to include in the brief and to whom it should be sent for maximum impact.

The document, labeled 'Policy Brief,' has a descriptive, accurate title and cites the brief's source, which may be an organization, institution, or one or more authors. A brief has more credibility if it includes the author's credentials, title, affiliation, or other pertinent biographic information.

The first component in a policy brief is an executive summary, which, on one page, captures the issue, the failings of current policy, and what the brief recommends. The second component describes the problem, its context, and importance. It clearly lays out the problem's causes, magnitude, and impact, and provides a history – when and how the problem surfaced, key events, and what the current situation is. Informative headings, perhaps in the form of questions, break up the text.

Thirdly, the writer cites other policy options and explains why they are inadequate. A simple, easy to understand table or graph illustrates the main points. The fourth component is a clear policy recommendation that makes a detailed, convincing argument based on the author's research. It also suggests practical steps to correct the problem. Tables and graphs are appropriate here as well. Instead of providing an abundance of scientific information, a table should succinctly reference the author's other publications and any that support the policy recommendation.

The closing paragraph re-emphasizes the recommended actions, which the author can list in bullet form. A name and contact information at the end tell readers where they can go for more details.

Summary

Presenting or publishing study results is an important part of the research process because it makes scientific knowledge available to other investigators, has the potential to improve readers' lives, and attests to researchers' ethical behavior. Authors should first decide which audience they want to reach, then tailor their presentation or article accordingly. Whether the vehicle is a poster, article, oral presentation, press release, or policy brief, researchers must develop and refine the skills that enable them to communicate findings in a clear and meaningful way. Skilled communicators enhance their own and their institution's stature, and contribute to the public's well-being.

Note

1 www.ncbi.nlm.nih.gov/pubmed

References

Blackwell Publishing (Undated) *Best practice guidelines on publishing ethics: A publisher's perspective.* London: Blackwell Publishing.

Day, R.A. (2001) *How to write and publish a scientific paper.* Washington, D.C.: Organización Panamericana de la Salud.

Guimaraes, C.A. (2006) Structured abstracts: Narrative review. *Acta Cirurgica Brasileira,* **21**(4), 1–14.

Hansen, R. (2009) A barebones guide to writing successful press releases. Available at www.randallshansen.com/prhowto.html (Accessed May 5, 2009).

International Committee of Medical Journal Editors (2008) Uniform requirements for manuscripts submitted to biomedical journals: Writing and editing for biomedical publication. Available at www.ICMJE.org.

Kramer, M. (2005) *What is narrative?* Cambridge, MA: Harvard University.

Miller, J.E. (2007) Preparing and presenting effective research posters. *Health Services Research* **42**(1), 311–328.

Nakayama, T., Hirai, N., Yamazaki, S. & Maito, M. (2005) Adoption of structured abstracts by general medical journals: The case for a structured abstract. *Journal of the Medical Library Association* **93**(2), 237–242.

Quinterno, L. (2009) Tell them a story! The principles of narrative journalism. Available at cndls.georgetown.edu/applications/posterTool/index.cfm?fuseaction=poster. display&posterID=796 (Accessed web site May 5, 2009).

Stoller, B. (2009) How to write a great press release: A sample release template. Available at www.publicityinsider.com/release.asp (Accessed web site May 5, 2009).

Young, E. & Quinn, L. (2004) *The policy brief.* Local Government and Public Service Reform Initiative training material. Geneva: World Health Organization. Available at www.who.int/rpc/evipnet/PolicyBrief-described.pdf.

Chapter 21
Facilitating nursing research

Lauren S. Aaronson &
William L. Holzemer

Introduction

Research is not a solitary enterprise. Like the often-stated wisdom that it takes a village to raise a child, it takes a community to facilitate research. This community of scholars – peers with whom one shares ideas in solving ever-present dilemmas during research, and who provide the intellectual environment in which science thrives – includes the organization or institution where the investigator works. The university, school of nursing, or hospital or other clinical facility must provide the necessary infrastructure to support investigators.

Resource centers for nursing research

Academic and clinical settings place high value on conducting research and integrating the results into practice. To accomplish this, they must become a resource center for information, offer expertise in research methodology, and support pre- and post-grant award activities. Since the early 1970s in the USA, amid the expansion of doctoral education in nursing, many schools of nursing have established an office of research to provide these services to faculty. In addition, some clinical settings, such as hospitals and home care agencies, have established centers of excellence to support nursing research and evidence-based practice. The goal of such centers is to create 'one-stop shopping' for the research-related knowledge, skills, support, and management that faculty and clinical staff need.

Resource centers for nursing research create an investigator-friendly and supportive atmosphere of open access to all types of information, policies, and rules regarding research activities and grants.

Research information

The main function of resource centers is to serve as a fountain of knowledge about the many different types of sources for research funding, including national governmental agencies, state or provincial agencies, non-profit organizations such as the International Red Cross, pharmaceutical companies, and industry. Newsletters from a number of sources inform the centers about funding opportunities – information they must bring to the attention of researchers.

Examples of national entities that fund medical and health-related research are the Nursing Research Fund[1] at the Canadian Health Services Research Foundation and the Canadian Institutes of Health Research.[2] The National Science Council[3] in Taiwan also funds nursing research (Yin et al. 2000). Although more than 70% of published nursing research in England is unfunded (Rafferty et al. 2003), support is available from the National Health Service and the quality research program at the Higher Education Funding Council for England[4] (Centre for Policy in Nursing Research et al. 2001). The Australian government provides support through the National Health and Medical Research Council,[5] in the Department of Health and Ageing, and through the Australian Research Council,[6] in the Department of Education, Science, and Training. Nurse investigators in Queensland also can apply for funding from the Queensland Nursing Council.[7] Many US investigators receive funding from the National Institute of Nursing Research[8] at the National Institutes of Health (NIH) – considered a model of nursing-related research support – and other institutes within the NIH.

Often, a university-wide grant support office can help investigators find potential funders. Some institutions tailor this service to particular needs. Two especially useful websites are the US government's www.grants.gov and the Grantsmanship Center's www.tgci.com/funding.shtml. Grants.gov, established in 2002, is a storehouse of information on more than 1000 federal grant programs. The Grantsmanship Center, founded in 1972 to train non-profit and government agencies, offers free online information about public and private grants available locally (searchable by state), nationally, and internationally. Each year, it also offers more than 150 workshops for researchers and non-profit organizations.

Although these websites are easy to search, results may be more fruitful if investigators enlist the help of resource center staff who are familiar with the sites' capabilities. A center may be willing to search databases on an investigator's behalf, after it meets with him or her to determine the nature of a proposed study. On their own, investigators can at least learn about available funding sources.

It is important to identify potential funders early in the research process because, in addition to meeting application deadlines and eligibility requirements, and wading through instructions for filling out the necessary forms, applicants must determine if their research focus aligns with the focus and goals specified in a funder's call for proposals or announcements about grants. Principal investigators must convince a funder that their proposal is exactly the kind of project it is seeking. A proposal that does not meet the basic eligibility requirements or does not fall within the parameters of a call for proposals or funding program is a waste of everyone's time.

Each grant opportunity has unique policies and procedures governing applications. The resource center should be knowledgeable about these, as well as the university's or clinical entity's. Universities have their own policies and procedures governing applications submitted to the local committee that reviews grants for the protection of human and animal subjects. It is very helpful to have all of this information available in one location.

Resource centers keep samples of many different types of research grant applications on file, including grants for training and post-doctoral fellowships and grants from national governmental agencies and pharmaceutical companies. For novice grant applicants, such samples are extremely helpful. Centers need to have funders' permission to make the samples available.

Some centers also keep a file of study instruments that the university's faculty and staff use in research. The file, in paper or electronic form, may include instrument descriptions, copies, manuals, permission requirements, and samples of studies in which investigators applied an instrument.

Many nursing studies include laboratory values and self-report measures, or biomarkers. Some resource centers keep a file on biomarkers in nursing research and may arrange for investigators to speak with experts about them – for example, about the potential relationship between stress and cortisol levels or between quality of life and HIV viral load. A center may not have the internal expertise for this purpose, but it can develop a referral list and possibly provide the financial support that would enable faculty and staff to consult with outside experts.

Some centers maintain listings of faculty and staff interests. The listings help new faculty and graduate students locate investigators who have similar interests, and are a public relations resource for a center when it describes the institution's research activities. Many universities post the listings on their website so student applicants and potential faculty recruits can learn about the type of research conducted in particular settings.

Given the explosion in academic nursing, including new PhD programs, it is somewhat surprising that little has been published about ways to support and facilitate research, and to help nurse investigators compete for funding. Articles that address support for research productivity, primarily from a US perspective, include those by Conn et al. (2005), Crain and Broome (2000), Froman et al. (2003), and Yoon et al. (2002). Yoon et al. reported on a survey of US colleges and schools of nursing with doctoral programs about the support they provide. The other articles describe how a college or nursing school has internally supported and promoted research.

Methodology expertise

The second major focus of resource centers is to provide expertise in research methodology – how to prepare grant applications, analyze data, and write up study results. Center staff should have expertise in both quantitative and qualitative methods. For quantitative research, the expertise often is in study design, development of psychometrics or instruments, data management, data analysis, sampling, surveys, power analyses, and many other research components. For qualitative research, expertise includes how to use software for textual analysis of interview or focus group data.

A center should also be knowledgeable about technology for audio and video recording of observations. Web-based surveys, electronic data entry systems, and computer-assisted interviewing are becoming increasingly common technologies for gathering information. Faculty and staff need expertise on how to leverage, select, implement, and manage these new technologies.

Many resource centers offer short courses on research methods. The courses may last 1–2 hours and concentrate on, for example, a software upgrade, or they may last several days and focus on a topic such as multilevel statistical modeling.

Yet another key function of resource centers is peer review of grant applications before submission. If an office cannot conduct peer reviews itself, it should be able to facilitate them. Investigators should enlist one or more colleagues or mentors to review their grant applications, as numerous workshops, seminars, courses, articles, and grant-writing presentations have recommended. Neither peer review nor acceptance of reviewers' comments or recommendations is required, unlike the peer review associated with scientific papers, but researchers who take advantage of this process will likely submit a stronger proposal.

A cultural change may be in order if institutions or their investigators do not actively conduct peer reviews of grant applications and other work. Although changing the culture is never easy, it is necessary if an institution hopes to move toward a robust research program. The first step is to start with investigators who are receptive to peer review. When they tell colleagues about its value and their own positive experience, others will become receptive, too. Over time, peer review will become part of the institutional culture. One way to foster acceptance of peer review is to begin with senior investigators, who are more comfortable with critiques and may serve as models for less-experienced colleagues.

Establishing a peer-review norm is healthy for all aspects of research – from developing ideas into studies through preparation of findings for publication. Many researchers undergo reviews before they submit their manuscripts to journals, by asking colleagues for an informal critique. A resource center can help by connecting authors with willing reviewers.

An especially helpful approach is critiques of grant applications in group sessions. After all reviewers have read a proposal, the group convenes and discusses everyone's concerns and suggestions. Consequently, the principal investigator is not left pondering whose comments should be heeded if suggestions by two or more colleagues differ; rather, the group can collectively mull reactions and thoughts, then agree on the best direction. This often generates new ideas for strengthening the original proposal. Reviewers with formal review experience for major funders, such as the NIH, are valuable contributors to group sessions. The goal is to craft a proposal that the larger scientific community will understand and value.

Group peer review requires a substantial commitment by reviewers and the principal investigator, who must prepare a proposal well in advance of the deadline and account for this step in planning the grant application. The principal investigator also must be receptive to critiques of something he or she has spent many months developing. It takes a strong ego to endure this process, but researchers who have done so attest to its tremendous value, which far exceeds the value of individual feedback.

Group sessions are most valuable when they function as mock reviews, focusing on the criteria established by the targeted grant-maker. The applicant should sit in the room and simply listen for at least the first hour, as if he or she were not present, while the first and subsequent reviewers critique the grant proposal. This is difficult without feeling compelled to justify the proposal or respond to questions. However, a mock review simulates a real review, which the applicant will not attend. The application must speak for itself.

The resource center director facilitates group sessions by identifying potential reviewers within or outside the institution. Food or refreshments provided by the center or principal investigator is a small but welcome gesture of appreciation for participants' time and effort.

Grant funding is very competitive and often requires re-submission of a revised proposal, a time-consuming task that may greatly delay the start of research. Intense internal review not only improves the final product, but can also save considerable time by reducing the need for re-submissions.

Administration

In thinking about establishing a resource center, an institution must consider the entity's administrative responsibilities. Many schools of nursing in the USA have conferred the title 'associate dean of research' on the person who heads their center to denote the importance of its activities. In academic settings, such centers are sometimes led by someone who is not a nurse. The head of resource centers in clinical settings often receives the title 'director' or 'associate director.'

Establishing a resource center requires expertise, funding, and space – and, perhaps most importantly, an institutional commitment to science, nursing research, and evidence-based practice. It is not appropriate to mandate research by faculty members and then assign them 40 hours per week of classroom teaching. Without time in their work schedule, they cannot possibly conduct research.

Staffing a resource center is an evolutionary process. It may have a small staff initially, then grow as research activities and support efforts increase. Growth often occurs as grant funding for direct or indirect expenses becomes available. Yoon et al. (2002) found that the 56 research support offices they surveyed had an average of 4.2 ($\pm$ 2.5) full-time-equivalent staff members. The number and type of personnel will vary, depending on an organization's needs and stage of development and on the kind of support it provides. They may include a director, secretaries and clerical workers, statisticians, research assistants, grant administrators, accountants, individuals with information technology skills, and senior investigators serving as research consultants or mentors.

Resource centers commonly break down administrative research support into pre-award and post-award grants management activities; some centers are formally organized according to these two functions.

Pre-award grants management

Pre-award grants management involves everything from conceptually developing a grant proposal to writing and submitting it, and seeking related institutional approvals. Services may include helping faculty or staff review the literature and providing a grant writer to help prepare grant applications.

Most investigators, especially novices, greatly underestimate how long it will take to complete an application. The resource center needs to establish realistic timetables with clear deadlines the investigator must meet each step of the way. Developing a timetable usually begins by working backward from the application deadline to the present date, allowing ample time for the entire process. The Grant Application Process Planning Tool (Crain & Broome 2000) takes this approach in organizing the many steps between the conception of a research idea and submission of a grant application. The tool's three sections – preliminary development, proposal development and review, and application assembly and submission – identify specific tasks and actions, and recommend timeframes for accomplishing them.

In pre-award grants management, centers also may:

- Help a principal investigator assemble a research team. This might involve locating expertise outside the investigator's area of expertise and/or building an interdisciplinary team that has the necessary expertise and clinical contacts for a study.
- Provide grant-writing assistance and editing.
- Obtain all necessary approvals.
- Help the principal investigator develop a realistic budget within the funder's constraints. This includes meeting particular institutional requirements, such as budgeting for fringe benefits and vacations for faculty and staff.
- Ensure that a proposal complies with all relevant policies and with safeguards for protecting human or animal subjects.
- Conduct group peer-review sessions before a grant application is submitted. These sessions may serve an administrative as well as research purpose because some committees for the protection of human or animal subjects now require that all grant proposals undergo scientific scrutiny before the committee reviews a proposal, thereby ensuring that the study is significant and ethical.
- Submit grant applications electronically or deliver them physically by the deadline. Hard-copy applications may require up to 25 photocopies.

Typically, institutions rather than individual investigators tender grant applications and receive grant awards. An application from a college or university communicates its support and commitment by showing how much the institution will contribute to the project financially and otherwise, holding both the institution and investigator responsible for conducting the research, and making the institution accountable for meeting the funder's policy requirements and for submitting necessary reports and documents, including those related to expenses.

Given the complexity of the application process, an institution's imprimatur works to the benefit of most researchers, but it also means that applications must undergo institutional review before submission to funders. A resource center can help applicants leap this internal hurdle.

Post-award grants management

After grants are awarded, resource centers provide services to promote successful completion of funded studies. Typically, these services focus on fiscal and ethical activities related to the research rather the research itself. Activities include hiring personnel such as research assistants, setting up an institutional accounting system for the study, purchasing, tracking expenses, preparing monthly budget statements, estimating expenses over a 12-month period of the grant, preparing reports for the funder, and many other tasks.

Some resource centers are able to provide services more directly related to the mechanics of a study, such as managing data, preparing poster or slide presentations, or even preparing the manuscript. These post-award activities require significant additional resources and need to be accounted for in the principal investigator's grant application.

Conclusions

Promoting and facilitating nursing research is a collective enterprise. Therefore, these efforts require the commitment and support of the institution or organization where the research is based. Garnering commitment and support is easier at universities that explicitly make research a central mission, and where research may be an expectation, than it is at smaller colleges where the central mission is teaching. Many academics think this difference is primarily or exclusively related to the difference in teaching workloads in the two settings, but that is only part of the picture. An institution's culture and values also have an important role.

Some investigators at smaller institutions face overt opposition to conducting research, especially when resources are limited, because research does not fit the institution's teaching mission. In these cases, efforts to promote and facilitate research may be more successful if studies are related to teaching and professional practice. Such research is sorely needed and can make valuable contributions to nursing and health care generally, particularly if investigators share their study results with the community through scholarly publication.

Nurses who hope to become active researchers after obtaining a doctorate must seriously consider these issues when they assess various academic institutions as possible employers. This is not a difficult task. Universities and colleges openly promote and display their mission statements, and administrators generally are willing to discuss the institution's values and goals. Like applicants, administrators seek the best possible fit between those values and goals, and the needs of prospective faculty members. Other information is readily available as well. For example, one can enquire about the research activities of current faculty, not just those in nursing; the amount of external funding for this research; and whether there is a formal research administrative structure. If such a structure does not exist at a large institution, a nursing program is less likely to be able to successfully support and facilitate robust research. At a minimum, the institution should have an office responsible for submitting extramural grant applications, and an office or mechanisms to provide financial accounting to the funder on behalf of the investigator and to meet other regulatory requirements. This is particularly important when the funder requires compliance with rules and regulations regarding issues such as drug-free workplaces, equal opportunity employment practices, and assistance with the formal financial accounting between it and the recipient institution.

Larger clinical facilities may actively support and promote research and, like larger colleges and universities, cite research in their mission statement. If other health professionals at that facility are conducting research, it is a sign the facility would also be open to research by nurses. An active nursing research program and demonstrated use of study results in practice are often factors that help US hospitals achieve 'magnet status.' This coveted distinction, based on the strength and quality of a facility's nursing component, is awarded by the American Nurses' Credentialing Center, an affiliate of the American Nurses Association.[9]

This chapter described how resource centers support and facilitate research, and some of the related organizational, setting, and cultural issues. While this task is easier at larger institutions that have a research mission, others can adopt or adapt many of the same mechanisms. For example, smaller clinical facilities might focus on how they can conduct site-specific studies to address health care concerns or problems their affiliated institution has identified. Regardless of the setting, the organizational culture must value peer review and make it part of routine practice if science and research are to thrive.

Given that obtaining funding is a critical task for nurse scientists and other researchers, this chapter also explained how resource centers are a key asset when it comes to grant applications, as they can provide many different resources and services to investigators. Resource centers take many forms, begin small, and grow as activities and needs grow. Their first steps may be to sponsor research seminars or discussion groups for nurses regarding patient or nursing care problems in need of solutions.

Developing a resource center takes time and the dedicated support of those whose skills and experience will help investigators complete the research mission. These efforts can greatly benefit the institution when investigators receive the extramural financial support they need to complete their studies. Resource centers in academic or service settings are resource-intensive but absolutely necessary for successful research. Center leaders must have mentorship skills that will help young researchers become independent scientists. Even the most experienced scientist often needs assistance with pre-grant and post-grant award management, as the policies and procedures governing grant applications and the proper conduct of research are constantly changing.

In summary, resource centers should be designed to operate as centers of excellence.

Notes

1 www.chsrf.ca/nursing_research_fund/index_e.php
2 www.cihr-irsc.gc.ca/e/193.html
3 web1.nsc.gov.tw
4 www.hefce.ac.uk
5 www.nhmrc.gov.au
6 www.arc.gov.au
7 www.qnc.qld.gov.au/home/content.aspx?content=Grants,_Scholarships_&_Bursaries/
   Research_Grants
8 www.ninr.nih.gov
9 For more information about magnet status, see www.nursingadvocacy.org/faq/
   magnet.html.

References

Centre for Policy in Nursing Research, CHEMS Consulting, Higher Education Consultancy Group, Research Forum for Allied Health Professions (2001) *Promoting research in nursing and the allied health professions*. Bristol: Higher Education Funding Council.

Conn, V., Porter, R., McDaniel, R., Rantz, M. & Maas, M. (2005) Building research productivity in an academic setting. *Nursing Outlook* **53**(5), 224–231.

Crain, H. & Broome, M. (2000) Tool for planning the grant application process. *Nursing Outlook* **48**(6), 288–293.

Froman, R., Hall, A., Shah, A., Bernstein, J. & Galloway, R. (2003) A methodology for supporting research and scholarship. *Nursing Outlook* **51**(2), 84–89.

Rafferty, A., Traynor, M., Thompson, D., Ilott, I. & White, E. (2003) Research in nursing, midwifery, and the allied health professions. *British Medical Journal* **326**(7394), 833–834.

Yin, T., Hsu, N., Tsai, S., Wang, B., Shaw, F., Shih, F., et al. (2000) Priority-setting for nursing research in the Republic of China. *Journal of Advanced Nursing* **32**(1), 19–27.

Yoon, S., Wolfe, S., Yucha, C. & Tsai, P. (2002) Research support by doctoral-granting colleges/schools of nursing. *Journal of Professional Nursing* **18**(1), 16–21.

Part 7
Translating research to practice

Chapter 22
Information and communication technology infrastructure for evidence-based practice

Suzanne Bakken, Leanne M. Currie &
Ritamarie John

Introduction

An information and communication technology infrastructure provides an important foundation for evidence-based practice. Given that nursing practice is a rich source of knowledge development, such an infrastructure and its components must not only support the application of evidence *to* practice, but also build evidence *from* practice.

This chapter provides an overview of the components of an information and communication technology infrastructure for evidence-based practice. It also explains how nurses use the infrastructure.

Infrastructure for evidence-based practice

Components of an information and community technology infrastructure that supports evidence-based practice include:

- Data acquisition methods and user interfaces;
- Standards that facilitate health care data exchange among various information systems;
- Data repositories;

- Data mining techniques;
- Digital sources of evidence;
- Communication technologies; and
- Informatics competencies (Bakken 2001; Institute of Medicine 2004).

The following sections briefly describe each of these.

Acquisition methods and interfaces

Because clinical data entry is time-consuming, error-prone, and expensive (Shortliffe & Cimino 2006), it is important to optimize interfaces between computers and users. Speech recognition technology is well-accepted by clinicians and successful in structured domains such as radiology, but it is rarely used in nursing practice. Consequently, to record narrative information, nurses typically use multiple input devices, such as a mouse, keyboard, and touch screen. While using a mouse or stylus to select items from a list is appropriate for structured data, often typing is also necessary to create a narrative detailing the nuances of a particular clinical situation. Sub-optimal user interfaces can result in inefficient data entry and errors due to issues such as greater cognitive demands on the user (Horsky et al. 2004, 2005). In addition, to reduce the burden of data entry and optimize evidence-based practice, data should be re-used for multiple purposes. For example, a coagulation study result from the laboratory can be re-used in a system that assesses for risk of fall-related injury and provides evidence-based practice recommendations based on a set of rules. To enable re-use, data must be represented in a manner that enables computer systems to process and exchange the information.

Data exchange standards

Standards support the creation of information technology systems that can exchange data and understand them, and re-use data for multiple purposes, such as evidence-based practice, quality management, and patient safety. Many types of data exchange standards, including those for messaging and clinical guidelines, are relevant to nursing and must be tested to ensure that they support nursing practice (Danko et al. 2003; Dykes et al. 2003; Goossen et al. 2004; Choi et al. 2006). Standards related to representation of nursing concepts in information systems are specific to nursing and therefore especially important. These include standardized terminologies and reference terminology models.

Decades of research have resulted in a set of core nursing terminologies that represent the practice of nursing, make it easier to integrate nursing data into information systems (including electronic health records), and can be used for evidence-based practice, quality management, patient safety, and nursing research (Beyea 2000; Johnson et al. 2000; McCloskey & Bulechek 2000; Martin 2004; NANDA International 2008).[1] In addition, nurse researchers have demonstrated the utility of non-nursing terminologies for describing nursing practice (Griffith & Robinson 1993; Henry et al. 1994; Bakken et al. 2000a) and have led efforts to integrate nursing concepts into broader health care terminologies, such as the Logical Observation Identifiers, Names, and Codes (LOINC) database and the Systematized Nomenclature of Medicine (SNOMED) clinical terms (Bakken et al. 2002b; Matney et al. 2003). Of key importance at the international level has been the development and implementation of the International Classification of Nursing Practice, led by the International Council of Nurses (Coenen et al. 2001a, 2001b; Ehnfors et al. 2004; Hardiker et al. 2006). Table 22.1 summarizes these standard terminologies, their application in nursing, and other related factors.

Because nurses use multiple standardized terminologies in practice, investigators have conducted substantial research on transforming organized lists of nursing diagnoses and interventions into reference terminology models (RTMs) for computers (Hardiker & Rector 1998, 2001; Ozbolt 2000a, 2000b, 2003a; Hardiker et al. 2002; Choi et al. 2005). Less research has been carried out on transforming goals and outcomes (Bakken et al. 2000b, 2002a; Ozbolt 2003b). RTMs facilitate mapping among various nursing terminologies and enable computers to process terms for purposes such as decision support for evidence-based practice and aggregation of data from different terminologies. The culmination of this work was the development of an international standard that specifies RTMs for nursing diagnoses and interventions (Bakken et al. 2004b; International Standards Organization 2003). This standard has been tested in numerous studies and is being refined (Bakken et al. 2000b, 2002b, 2005; Hwang et al. 2003; Moss et al. 2003).

Even in the absence of information systems, standardized nursing terminologies have a vital role in communication about nursing practice and should be incorporated into paper documentation, such as critical pathways, flow sheets, and nursing care plans. This paper-based mechanism applies evidence to practice and is an interim step toward electronic nursing documentation and, by means of data mining, the building of evidence from practice.

Data repositories

Data repositories vary in terms of purpose, size, and the technologies for implementing them. Clinical data repositories, which often comprise a set of databases that relate to each other, collect patient care information from diverse sources and are designed to store and retrieve information about individual patients. Such repositories are essential in enabling evidence-based practice for a specific patient because the clinical context is usually spread across a variety of data sources (Bakken et al. 2004a). In some instances, data from the clinical data repository are reorganized in a clinical data warehouse. Although a warehouse typically contains information similar to that in a repository, it is optimized for long-term storage, retrieval, and analysis of aggregate patient data. Therefore, through a variety of data mining techniques, the warehouse can have a significant role in generating evidence from practice.

A stand-alone, project-specific database may be able to support smaller evidence-based-practice projects. However, unlike a clinical data repository, it will not benefit from automated acquisition of data from other information systems, so it may not fully capture clinical context in an efficient way. For example, a patient's medications would need to be re-entered into a project-specific database; they could not be transferred from the pharmacy's system. In addition, data stored only in a project-specific database are unlikely to inform clinical care beyond information related to the project. With appropriate protection

Table 22.1 Standardized terminologies and their use in nursing.

Terminology	Contents	Recognized by American Nurses Association	Included in Unified Medical Language System	Registered with Health Level 7	Included in SNOMED	Availability
Nursing-specific						
CCC*	Nursing diagnoses, interventions, outcomes, goals	✓	✓	✓	✓	Public domain
International Classification of Nursing Practice	Problems, interventions, outcomes	✓	✓	✓	✓	License
Omaha System	Problems, interventions, outcomes	✓	✓	✓	✓	Public domain
NANDA Taxonomy	Nursing diagnoses	✓	✓	✓	✓	License
Nursing Interventions Classification	Nursing interventions	✓	✓	✓	✓	License
Nursing Outcomes Classification	Patient/client outcomes	✓	✓	✓	✓	License
Patient Care Data Set	Patient problems, care goals, care orders	✓	✓	✓		Only at Vanderbilt University
Perioperative Nursing Data Set	Nursing diagnoses, interventions, patient outcomes	✓	✓	✓	✓	License
Not nursing-specific						
LOINC	Vital signs, obstetric measurements, clinical assessment scales, research instruments	✓	✓	✓	Laboratory LOINC only	Copyrighted, but free for use
SNOMED clinical terms	MD/RN diagnoses, health care interventions, procedures, findings, substances, organisms, events	✓	✓	✓	—	License

CCC, Clinical Care Classification; LOINC, Logical Observation Identifiers, Names, and Codes; SNOMED, Systematized Nomenclature of Medicine.
* Formerly the Home Health Care Classification.

of privacy and confidentiality, integration of clinical and research data can reduce the time it takes to translate research evidence into practice.

Data mining

Data mining techniques, also known as 'knowledge discovery in databases,' include traditional statistical approaches, artificial intelligence methods, and natural language processing. In the health care context, data mining typically focuses on re-using information collected during the course of care for other purposes, such as quality management, patient safety, and clinical research. Data mining has been used less frequently to build evidence from practice.

Goodwin et al. (2003) have applied a variety of data mining techniques – logistic regression, neural networks, classification and regression trees, inductive algorithms, and fuzzy logic – to practice data to discover predictors of pre-term birth. Abbott et al. (1998) applied the Minimum Data Set, a tool that long-term care facilities use to assess residents, to discover predictors of admission to acute care from long-term care. Hyun et al. (2009) explored the ability of natural language processing to extract, from nursing narratives, data related to chemotherapy side effects, pain management, and nosocomial infections.

Although data mining is under-utilized as a way to generate evidence from practice, work to date suggests it has potential value for this purpose. Capturing nursing data in electronic format is an essential prerequisite to applying data mining techniques.

Digital sources of evidence

The web and powerful search engines have improved access to a broad variety of digital sources of evidence. These sources have expanded beyond the primary bibliographic literature to include systematic reviews, meta-analyses, and synopses, such as clinical practice guidelines and standards of care, which are aimed at facilitating evidence-based practice. The challenge is matching information needs to high-quality sources in an efficient and clinically relevant manner, not just finding information. One approach is to create context-specific links that provide access to institutional and external sources of evidence from within a clinical information system – for example, a link from the medication administration record to evidence-based patient education materials. A number of studies have shown that such approaches are useful (Cimino 2006; Maviglia et al. 2006).

Communication technologies

Communication networks, such as the Internet, intranets, and cellular networks, and the devices associated with them, are essential for enabling access to digital sources of evidence at the point of care. Increasingly, caregivers are using personal digital assistants, cell phones, tablet computers, and other mobile communication devices to shift the access point from stationary workstations to the point of care. Although the use of Web 2.0 tools – wikis, blogs, podcasts, vodcasts – in health care is in its infancy (Boulos et al. 2006), their potential role as mechanisms for building evidence from practice and applying evidence to practice is an exciting but relatively unexplored possibility.

Informatics competencies

Nurses must have sufficient knowledge and skills to be able to use evidence-based practice applications in information and communication technologies. Informatics competencies have been discussed in the nursing literature for nearly two decades, and there is greater interest now in ensuring that nursing graduates and practicing nurses have adequate competencies to meet the demands of various practice settings (Peterson & Gerdin-Jelger 1988; Grobe 1989; Carty & Rosenfeld 1998; Staggers et al. 2001, 2002). Much of the early research focused on basic computer skills for educational, clinical, and administrative purposes.

Information literacy, a prerequisite for evidence-based practice, includes knowing when a need for information exists, identifying the information that addresses a problem or issue, finding and evaluating the information, organizing it, and using it effectively to address the problem or issue (American Library Association 1989; National Forum on Information Literacy 1998). In a national survey of nurses, Tanner et al. (2004) found that although most respondents had regular information needs, more than half never searched electronic databases, evaluated research reports, or used research results in practice. Other findings suggest that nurses lack adequate training in the use of tools to locate evidence on which to base their practice (Pravikoff et al. 2005).

Staggers et al. (2001, 2002) have carried out extensive research on defining informatics competency for nursing. They published a set of informatics competencies at four levels of practice: beginning nurse, experienced nurse, informatics specialist, and informatics innovator. There has been little research to document how well nurses meet these competencies, which go beyond computer and information literacy to include knowledge and skills regarding clinical applications that support evidence-based practice (McNeil et al. 2004; Desjardins et al. 2005).

Sample infrastructure uses in nursing

The following examples illustrate how two institutions used their information and communication technology infrastructures to build and apply two different evidence-based-practice assessment tools. Table 22.2 shows the infrastructure components.

Fall and injury risk assessment

Although there are a number of validated instruments for assessing the risk of falls, investigators at New York Presbyterian Hospital (NYPH) wanted to create one that would be tailored to the types of patients the hospital serves and, unlike other instruments, would predict the risk of a fall-related injury. The research team built evidence from practice by conducting a retrospective, case–control study to determine the fall and injury risk among NYPH's medical and surgical patients. It proposed a tool called the Fall-Injury Risk Assessment, which included five fall-related predictors (fall[s] in the past 7 days, use of sedatives or hypnotics, male gender, impaired cognition, and impaired condition) and two injury-related predictors (risk for bleeding and risk for fracture) (Currie et al. 2004). Each predictor was weighted based on NYPH data.

Table 22.2 Information and communication infrastructure tools at two institutions.

Component	Fall-Injury Risk Assessment (New York Presbyterian Hospital)	Mobile Decision Support for Advanced Practice Nursing (Columbia University School of Nursing)
Data acquisition methods and user interfaces	Clinician data entry into one of two clinical information systems augments data acquired from clinical data repository	Nurse practitioner students enter assessment and care-plan data, which are transferred among system modules to support a system-generated diagnosis and a tailored plan of care
Data exchange standards	Standardized terminologies: UMLS and the LOINC database	Standardized terminologies: ICD-9-CM, CPT Codes, CCC System, SNOMED clinical terms
Data repositories	Institutional data repository and clinical data warehouse	Project-specific access to database
Data mining techniques	Traditional statistical methods for extracting clinical data to determine fall-injury predictors among patients at New York Presbyterian Hospital	N/A
Digital sources of evidence or knowledge	Multiple sources of fall-injury risk assessment and management are represented as concepts and integrated into an institutional data dictionary	Multiple sources of depression guidelines are decomposed, represented in a project-specific knowledge base, and integrated into a five-part plan of care
Communication technologies	Internet	Internet, cellular network, cell phones, personal digital assistants
Informatics competencies	Included in general communication and information system training	15-hour course on informatics competencies for evidence-based practice and patient safety, and 1 hour of application-specific training

CCC, Clinical Care Classification; CPT, Current Procedural Terminology; ICD-9-CM, International Classification of Diseases, Clinical Modification; LOINC, Logical Observation, Identifiers, Names, and Codes; SNOMED, Systematized Nomenclature of Medicine; UMLS, Unified Medical Language System.

Administrative and practice experts then evaluated the instrument and suggested revisions that would improve its usability in practice. Subsequently, NYPH deployed an automated Fall-Injury Risk Assessment with tailored, evidence-based safety measures in two clinical information systems. Nurses routinely use the instrument, and studies to evaluate its impact on fall and injury rates are ongoing. The hospital is taking a similar approach, based on statistical data mining, to design a Fall-Injury Risk Assessment tool for behavioral health settings.

Data are represented in the institutional data dictionary using Unified Medical Language System and LOINC codes. Data such as age and gender are pre-populated in the Fall-Injury Risk Assessment with data from the clinical data repository. Clinicians enter data related to other risk factors at the time they assess risk. The infrastructure supports the iterative cycle of building evidence from practice and applying evidence to practice.

Decision support for nursing students

Columbia University designed a tool called Mobile Decision Support for Advanced Practice Nursing (MODS-APN) to aid nurse practitioner students at its School of Nursing (Bakken et al. 2006). The students are randomly assigned to receive decision support via a personal digital assistant (PDA) for screening and managing tobacco use, obesity, or depression.

The first of two key tasks for the project team that developed this tool was selecting the evidence upon which the decision support would be based. One clinical practice guideline provided the primary evidence for smoking cessation and another provided the primary evidence for obesity management in adults (Fiore et al. 2000; National Institutes of Health et al. 2000). However, because there was no single guideline for adult or pediatric depression screening and management, the team used multiple sources of evidence (Sharp & Lipsky 2002; US Preventive Services Task Force 2002; Institute for Clinical Systems Improvement 2004; University of Michigan Health System 2004; Hamrin & Pachler 2005; Richmond & Rosen 2005). It selected the two-item and four-item surveys in the Patient Health Questionnaire for adult depression screening because of the questionnaire's broad use in other primary care depression projects. Choosing a standardized assessment for pediatric screening across ages 8–17 was especially challenging (John et al. 2007). After a careful literature review, discussion among team members, and consultation with internal and external experts, the team selected the Short Mood and Feeling Questionnaire to measure 'risk for mood disorder' rather than an instrument for longer-term diagnosis (Angold et al. 1995; Myers & Winters 2002; Dahlberg et al. 2005). It added four questions – two related to family history of depression and two related to suicide (Elliott & Smiga 2003; Apter & King 2006).

The second major task was integrating the evidence from multiple sources about managing depression into a suitable format for MODS-APN. (The team used similar methods for management and screening of tobacco use and obesity.) After the team assembled the pediatric depression evidence, it decomposed the evidence into the five-part nurse practitioner plan of care – diagnostics, procedures, prescriptions, patient teaching, and referrals – which students learn about in the clinical curriculum. This template reminds students about the elements of evidence-based practice for pediatric depression and enables them to document each one.

The PDA-based clinical log provides decision support in three ways. First, the student receives a reminder during the initial encounter to screen for these conditions. Second, he or she sees an age-appropriate, standardized screening assessment to be completed while interviewing the patient. Third, the decision support system automatically generates a diagnosis based on the assessment score. A five-part plan of care tailored to the diagnosis, such as no risk for mood disorder or suicide, at risk for mood disorder, or at risk for mood disorder and suicide, provides a template to guide the delivery and documentation of care. An algorithm developed by the project team and implemented in AppForge software for the PDA drives these actions (John et al. 2007).

MODS-APN acquires data primarily through user data entry; there are touch-screen radio buttons and pull-down menus for this purpose. It does not acquire data from external information systems, but rather transfers them from one part of the application to another. For example, a patient's age and depression-screening score tailor the five parts in the plan of care presented to the student for action. Table 22.2 lists the standardized terminologies that MODS-APN uses to represent content. The architecture includes a data repository and, in addition to PDAs, supports mobile devices such as cell phones.

Unlike the Fall-Injury Risk Assessment, MODS-APN is not integrated into a larger clinical information system. A randomized controlled trial is evaluating its efficacy. If MODS-APN is found to improve caregivers' adherence to guideline recommendations, Columbia University's information and communication infrastructure will facilitate its integration into other information systems.

Conclusions

The rate of knowledge development continues to escalate and health care settings are busier than ever. As a result, nurses are continually challenged to provide care that is consistent with the best available evidence. An information and communication technology infrastructure is an important foundation for building evidence from practice and applying evidence to practice. Some components of the infrastructure, such as standardized terminologies and digital sources of evidence, have been the focus of substantial nursing research. Although applying data mining tools to build evidence from practice and to assess the effect of evidence on practice is still in its infancy, it is highly relevant and warrants further attention.

Infrastructure tools for evidence-based practice cannot achieve optimal impact if their intended users do not have the necessary information literacy and informatics competencies. Therefore, competency-based training should accompany the implementation of evidence-based-practice tools.

Note

1 See also Saba, V.K. Clinical care classification system. Available at www. sabacare.com.

References

Abbott, P.A., Quirolgico, S., Manchand, R., Canfield, K. & Adya, M. (1998) Can the US Minimum Data Set be used for predicting admissions to acute care facilities? *MedInfo* **9**, 1318–1321.

American Library Association (1989) *Presidential Committee on Information Literacy. Final report*. Chicago: American Library Association.

Angold, A., Costello, E. & Messer, S. (1995) Development of a short questionnaire for use in epidemiological studies of depression in children and adolescents: Factor composition and structure across development. *International Journal of Methods in Psychiatric Research* **5**, 237–249.

Apter, A. & King, R.A. (2006) Management of the depressed, suicidal child or adolescent. *Child and Adolescent Psychiatric Clinics of North America* **15**(4), 999–1013.

Bakken, S. (2001) An informatics infrastructure is essential for evidence-based practice. *Journal of the American Medical Informatics Association* **8**(3), 199–201.

Bakken, S., Chen, E., Choi, J., Currie, L.M., Lee, N.J., Roberts, W.D., et al. (2006) Mobile decision support for advanced practice nurses. *Studies in Health Technology and Informatics* **122**, 1002.

Bakken, S., Cimino, J.J., Haskell, R., Kukafka, R., Matsumoto, C., Chan, G.K., et al. (2000a) Evaluation of the clinical LOINC (Logical Observation Identifiers, Names, and Codes) semantic structure as a terminology model for standardized assessment measures. *Journal of the American Medical Informatics Association* **7**(6), 529–538.

Bakken, S., Cashen, M.S., Mendonca, E.A., O'Brien, A. & Zieniewicz, J. (2000b) Representing nursing activities within a concept-oriented terminological system: Evaluation of a type definition. *Journal of the American Medical Informatics Association* **7**(1), 81–90.

Bakken, S., Cimino, J.J. & Hripcsak, G. (2004a) Promoting patient safety and enabling evidence-based practice through informatics. *Medical Care* **42**(2 Suppl), II49–II56.

Bakken, S., Coenen, A. & Saba, V. (2004b) ISO reference technology model: Nursing diagnosis and action models look to testing for practical application. *Healthcare Informatics* **21**(9), 52.

Bakken, S., Hyun, S., Friedman, C. & Johnson, S.B. (2005) ISO reference terminology models for nursing: Applicability for natural language processing of nursing narratives. *International Journal of Medical Informatics* **74**(7–8), 615–622.

Bakken, S., Warren, J.J., Casey, A., Konicek, D., Lundberg, C. & Pooke, M. (2002a) Information model and terminology model issues related to goals. *AMIA Annual Symposium Proceedings* 17–21.

Bakken, S., Warren, J.J., Lundberg, C., Casey, A., Correia, C., Konicek, D., et al. (2002b) An evaluation of the usefulness of two terminology models for integrating nursing diagnosis concepts into SNOMED Clinical Terms. *International Journal of Medical Informatics* **68**(1–3), 71–77.

Beyea, S. (2000) Perioperative data elements: Interventions and outcomes. *Association of Operating Room Nurses Journal* **71**(2), 344–353.

Boulos, M.N., Maramba, I. & Wheeler, S. (2006) Wikis, blogs and podcasts: A new generation of Web-based tools for virtual collaborative clinical practice and education. *BMC Medical Education* **6**, 41.

Carty, B. & Rosenfeld, P. (1998) From computer technology to information technology: Findings from a national study of nursing education. *Computers in Nursing* **16**(5), 259–265.

Choi, J., Jenkins, M.L., Cimino, J.J., White, T.M. & Bakken, S. (2005) Toward semantic interoperability in home health care: Formally representing OASIS items for integration into a concept-oriented terminology. *Journal of the American Medical Informatics Association* **12**(4), 410–417.

Choi, J., Sapp, J. & Bakken, S. (2006) Encoding a depression screening guideline using GLIF. *Studies in Health Technology and Informatics* **122**, 905–906.

Cimino, J.J. (2006) Use, usability, usefulness, and impact of an infobutton manager. *AMIA Annual Symposium Proceedings* 151–155.

Coenen, A., Marin, H.F., Park, H.A. & Bakken S. (2001a) Collaborative efforts for representing nursing concepts in computer-based systems: International perspectives. *Journal of the American Medical Informatics Association* **8**(3), 202–211.

Coenen, A., McNeil, B., Bakken, S., Bickford, C., Warren, J.J., American Nurses Association Committee on Nursing Practice Information Infrastructure (2001b) Toward comparable nursing data: American Nurses Association criteria for data sets, classification systems, and nomenclatures. *Computers in Nursing* **19**(6), 240–246.

Currie, L.M., Mellino, L.V., Cimino, J.J. & Bakken, S. (2004) Development and representation of a fall-injury risk assessment instrument in a clinical information system. *Studies in Health Technology and Informatics* **107**(Pt 1), 721–725.

Dahlberg, L.L., Toal, S.B., Swahn, M. & Behrens, C.B. (2005) *Measuring violence-related attitudes, behaviors, and influences among youths: A compendium of assessment tools*, 2nd Edn. Atlanta, GA: Centers for Disease Control and Prevention.

Danko, A., Kennedy, R., Haskell, R., Androwich, I.M., Button, P., Correia, C.M., et al. (2003) Modeling nursing interventions in the act class of HL7 RIM Version 3. *Journal of Biomedical Informatics* **36**(4–5), 294–303.

Desjardins, K.S., Cook, S.S., Jenkins, M. & Bakken, S. (2005) Effect of an informatics for evidence-based practice curriculum on nursing informatics competencies. *International Journal of Medical Informatics* **74**(11–12), 1012–1020.

Dykes, P.C., Currie, L.M. & Cimino, J.J. (2003) Adequacy of evolving national standardized terminologies for interdisciplinary coded concepts in an automated clinical pathway. *Journal of Biomedical Informatics* **36**(4–5), 313–325.

Ehnfors, M., Coenen, A., Marin, H.F. & Prenkert, M. (2004) Translating the International Classification for Nursing Practice (ICNP): an experience from two countries. *Medinfo* **11**(Part 1), 502–505.

Elliott, G. & Smiga, S. (2003) Depression in the child and adolescent. *Pediatric Clinics of North America* **50**(5), 1093–1106.

Fiore, M.C., Bailey, W.C. & Cohen, S.J. (2000) *Clinical practice guideline: Treating tobacco use and dependence*. Rockville, MD: US Department of Health & Human Services.

Goodwin, L., VanDyne, M., Lin, S. & Talbert, S. (2003) Data mining issues and opportunities for building nursing knowledge. *Journal of Biomedical Informatics* **36**(4–5), 379–388.

Goossen, W.T., Ozbolt, J.G., Coenen, A., Park, H.A., Mead, C., Ehnfors, M., et al. (2004) Development of a provisional domain model for the nursing process for use within the Health Level 7 reference information model. *Journal of the American Medical Informatics Association* **11**(3), 186–194.

Griffith, H.M. & Robinson, K.R. (1993) Current Procedural Terminology (CPT) coded services provided by nurse specialists. *Image: Journal of Nursing Scholarship* **25**(3), 178–186.

Grobe, S. (1989) Nursing informatics competencies. *Methods of Information in Medicine* **28**(4), 267–269.

Hamrin, V. & Pachler, M.C. (2005) Child and adolescent depression: Review of the latest evidence-based treatments. *Journal of Psychosocial Nursing and Mental Health Services* **43**(1), 54–63.

Hardiker, N.R., Bakken, S., Casey, A., Hoy, D. (2002) Formal nursing terminology systems: A means to an end. *Journal of Biomedical Informatics* **35**(5–6), 298–305.

Hardiker, N.R., Casey, A., Coenen, A. & Konicek, D. (2006) Mutual enhancement of diverse terminologies. *AMIA Annual Symposium Proceedings* 319–323.

Hardiker, N.R. & Rector, A.L. (1998) Modeling nursing terminology using the GRAIL representation language. *Journal of the American Medical Informatics Association* **5**(1), 120–128.

Hardiker, N.R. & Rector, A.L. (2001) Structural validation of nursing terminologies. *Journal of the American Medical Informatics Association* **8**(3), 212–221.

Henry, S.B., Holzemer, W.L., Reilly, C.A. & Campbell, K.E. (1994) Terms used by nurses to describe patient problems: Can SNOMED III represent nursing concepts in the patient record? *Journal of the American Medical Informatics Association* **1**(1), 61–74.

Horsky, J., Kaufman, D.R. & Patel, V.L. (2004) Computer-based drug ordering: Evaluation of interaction with a decision-support system. *Medinfo* **11**(Pt 2), 1063–1067.

Horsky, J., Zhang, J. & Patel, V.L. (2005) To err is not entirely human: Complex technology and user cognition. *Journal of Biomedical Informatics* **38**(4), 264–266.

Hwang, J.I., Cimino, J.J. & Bakken, S. (2003) Integrating nursing diagnostic concepts into the medical entities dictionary using the ISO Reference Terminology Model for Nursing Diagnosis. *Journal of the American Medical Informatics Association* **10**(4), 382–388.

Hyun, S., Johnson, S. & Bakken, S. (2009) Exploring the ability of natural language processing to extract data from nursing narratives. *Computers, Informatics, Nursing.* July/August 27(4), 215–23.

Institute for Clinical Systems Improvement (2004) *Major depression in adults in primary care*. Bloomington, MN: Institute for Clinical Systems Improvement.

Institute of Medicine (2004) *Patient safety: achieving a new standard for care*. Washington, D.C.: Institute of Medicine.

International Standards Organization (2003) *Integration of a reference terminology model for nursing: FDIS*. Geneva: International Standards Organization.

John, R., Buschman, P., Chaszar, M., Honig, J., Mendonca, E. & Bakken, S. (2007) Development and evaluation of a PDA-based decision support system for pediatric depression screening. *Studies in Health Technology and Informatics* **129**(Pt 2), 1382–1386.

Johnson, M., Maas, M. & Moorhead, S. (Eds) (2000) *Nursing Outcomes Classification (NOC)*, 2nd Edn. St. Louis, MO: C.V. Mosby.

Martin, K.S. (2004) *The Omaha System: A key to practice, documentation, and information management*, 2nd Edn. St. Louis, MO: Elsevier.

Matney, S., Bakken, S. & Huff, S.M. (2003) Representing nursing assessments in clinical information systems using the Logical Observation Identifiers, Names, and Codes database. *Journal of Biomedical Informatics* **36**(4–5), 287–293.

Maviglia, S.M., Yoon, C.S., Bates, D.W. & Kuperman, G. (2006) KnowledgeLink: Impact of context-sensitive information retrieval on clinicians' information needs. *Journal of the American Medical Informatics Association* **13**(1), 67–73.

McCloskey, J.C. & Bulechek, G.M. (2000) *Nursing interventions classification*, 3rd Edn. St. Louis, MO: C.V. Mosby.

McNeil, B., Elfrink, V. & Pierce, S. (2004) Preparing student nurses, faculty and clinicians for 21st century informatics practice: Findings from a national survey of nursing education programs in the United States. *Studies in Health Technology and Informatics* **107**(Part 2), 903–907.

Moss, J., Coenen, A. & Mills, M.E. (2003) Evaluation of the draft international standard for a reference terminology model for nursing actions. *Journal of Biomedical Informatics* **36**(4–5), 271–278.

Myers, K. & Winters, N.C. (2002) Ten-year review of rating scales. II: Scales for internalizing disorders. *Journal of the American Academy of Child and Adolescent Psychiatry* **41**(6), 634–659.

NANDA International (2008) *Nursing diagnoses: Definitions and classification 2009–2011*. Philadelphia: NANDA International.

National Forum on Information Literacy (1998) *A progress report on information literacy: An update on the American Library Association Presidential Committee on Information Literacy: Final report*. San Jose, CA: National Forum on Information Literacy.

National Institutes of Health; National Heart, Lung, and Blood Institute; NHLBI Obesity Education Initiative; North American Association for the Study of Obesity (2000) *The practical guide. Identification, evaluation, and treatment of overweight and obesity in adults.* Bethesda, MD: National Institutes of Health.

Ozbolt, J. (2000a) Toward a reference terminology model for nursing: The 1999 Nursing Vocabulary Summit Conference. In V. Saba, R. Carr, W. Sermeus & P. Rocha (Eds), *7th International Congress of Nursing Informatics. One step beyond: The evolution of technology and nursing* (pp. 267–276). Auckland, New Zealand: Adis International.

Ozbolt, J. (2000b) Terminology standards for nursing: Collaboration at the summit. *Journal of the American Medical Informatics Association* **7**(6), 517–522.

Ozbolt, J. (2003a) The Nursing Terminology Summit Conferences: A case study of successful collaboration for change. *Journal of Biomedical Informatics* **36**(4–5), 362–374.

Ozbolt, J. (2003b) Reference terminology for therapeutic goals: A new approach. *AMIA Annual Symposium Proceedings* 504–508.

Peterson, H. & Gerdin-Jelger, U. (1988) *Preparing nurses for using information systems: Recommended informatics competencies.* New York: NLN Publications.

Pravikoff, D.S., Tanner, A.B. & Pierce, S.T. (2005) Readiness of US nurses for evidence-based practice. *American Journal of Nursing* **105**(9), 40–51.

Richmond, T.K. & Rosen, D.S. (2005) The treatment of adolescent depression in the era of the black box warning. *Current Opinion in Pediatrics* **17**(4), 466–472.

Sharp, L.K. & Lipsky, M.S. (2002) Screening for depression across the lifespan: A review of measures for use in primary care settings. *American Family Physician* **66**(6), 1001–1008.

Shortliffe, E.H. & Cimino, J. (Eds) (2006) *Biomedical informatics: Computer applications in health care and biomedicine*, 3rd Edn. New York: Springer Science.

Staggers, N., Gassert, C.A. & Curran, C. (2001) Informatics competencies for nurses at four levels of practice. *Journal of Nursing Education* **40**(7), 303–316.

Staggers, N., Gassert, C.A. & Curran, C. (2002) A Delphi study to determine informatics competencies for nurses at four levels of practice. *Nursing Research* **51**(6), 383–390.

Tanner, A., Pierce, S. & Pravikoff, D. (2004) Readiness for evidence-based practice: Information literacy needs of nurses in the United States. *Studies in Health Technology and Informatics* **107**(Part 2), 936–940.

University of Michigan Health System (2004) *University of Michigan depression guideline update*. Ann Arbor, MI: University of Michigan Health System.

US Preventive Services Task Force (2002) Screening for depression: Recommendations and rationale. *Annals of Internal Medicine* **136**(10):760–764.

Chapter 23
Translating research into practice

Cornelia Ruland

Introduction

Evidence-based practice (EBP) is a widely adopted model for good clinical care. In this model, health professionals are expected to demonstrate that they have applied the best available knowledge and advances gained from research findings, which requires access to valid, reliable, relevant, and updated information about the effects of health care interventions at the point of care. However, there is a considerable gap between existing evidence-based knowledge and its integration into clinical practice, for several reasons.

One reason is information overload. At least 2 million research articles are published annually in the medical and associated literature (Haines & Donald 2002). It is almost impossible for clinicians to keep up with research evidence, even in their own specialty. A second reason is that most clinicians do not have the time or evaluation skills to judge the relevance and quality of published research and its applicability to their own practice setting. Third, evidence-based information about the effectiveness of interventions is rarely available in a readily applicable format. Interventions may be effective under well-controlled conditions, but research reports hardly ever address the contextual details or practitioners' need to understand how to translate and implement evidence into the context of heterogeneous practices and patients (McDonald & Viehbeck 2007). Introducing new interventions usually requires organizational changes as well as adaptation to clinicians' workflow and the professional context.

The purpose of EBP is to support clinical practice decision-making. However, information that only addresses the effectiveness of interventions is usually not sufficient to inform clinicians about the best course of action. Clinical decisions often involve trade-offs between intervention alternatives; several options may be possible, each of them associated with different benefits and harms. Because the desire for particular outcomes varies among patients, treatment and care must be adjusted to the individual's values and experiences.

Therefore, appropriate clinical decision-making requires the consideration and sharing of two important aspects of knowledge. One is evidence about facts, such as the patient's diagnosis, symptoms, and problems; available treatment options; associated risks; and likely outcomes. The other aspect is information regarding what a patient values in terms of potential outcomes, given the patient's personal knowledge about, and experience living with, an illness and how it affects his or her life and well-being. For a clinician to be able to plan individualized, evidence-based care, this information needs to be elicited from patients and communicated to the clinician (Degner & Sloan 1992; Ruland 2005). Yet the EBP practice model pays little attention to the importance of patients' perspectives for appropriate treatment and care, and thus leaves out an important piece of evidence to support clinical decision-making.

While EBP primarily targets clinicians, patients also need evidence-based knowledge to manage their illness. They spend most of their time at home unsupervised by health care professionals. Extending EBP to the realm of patients' self-management of illness and providing them with evidence-based knowledge when and where they need it could significantly improve the safety and quality of patient care.

This chapter describes processes for overcoming barriers that inhibit the integration of EBP into clinical practice. These processes include systematic literature reviews in which evidence from multiple studies is synthesized and evaluated, and generating new evidence from both research and clinical practice. The chapter also describes models for shared decision-making that incorporate patients' perspectives, an important source of evidence, into clinical decisions.

Systematic literature reviews

Published research is an important source of information that helps policy-makers and clinicians make appropriate decisions. However, identifying findings that address clinicians' particular questions can be difficult. Furthermore, results from different studies may conflict, authors may neglect to interpret their findings in the context of previous research, and the quality of studies varies. Systematic literature reviews, a widely acknowledged method that involves synthesizing evidence from multiple studies about a topic, are considered to be the most reliable source of information regarding the effectiveness of health care interventions (Chalmers & Altmann 1995). They provide an overview of research in a specific area by finding, describing, rigorously evaluating, and summarizing the evidence in that area. Randomized controlled trials are the preferred type of study included in systematic reviews; researchers view them as having the lowest risk of bias. Such trials also enable reliable estimates of an intervention's effect.

Systematic reviews differ from other types of literature reviews in that they follow rigorous guidelines. Because clinicians rarely have the time and skills to conduct comprehensive reviews, a number of organizations specialize in them. Different organizations may perform different types of reviews. For example, the Cochrane Collaboration, an international not-for-profit, independent organization founded in 1993 by the British epidemiologist Archie Cochrane, specializes in systematic reviews of randomized controlled trials, although it takes other types of evidence into account if appropriate. The collaboration's major product is the Cochrane Database of Systematic Reviews, which are presented in a structured format that is relatively easy for non-experts to understand and which are published quarterly as part of the Cochrane Library.[1]

Other databases for evidence-based systematic reviews that are helpful to clinicians include the Turning Research Into Practice (TRIP) Database,[2] SUMsearch,[3] the Database of Abstracts of Reviews of Effects (DARE)[4] at the Centre for Reviews and Dissemination, BMJ Clinical Evidence,[5] and the National Institute for Health and Clinical Excellence (NICE).[6]

Systematic reviews are usually summarized in succinct reports to help readers evaluate the validity and implication of research findings. Most are available, and can be purchased, online. However, simply disseminating reviews does not change practice, and finding meaningful answers to clinical questions related to one's own practice is not always easy.

Clinicians who intend to apply evidence of an intervention's effectiveness need to consider all beneficial and harmful effects. They should explore variations in these effects – such as levels of risk and severity of illness – and the reasons for them, and whether the research findings need to be adjusted to local needs, which could lead to different results. In addition, readers must interpret the findings in terms of their applicability – that is, the extent to which the observed effects of studies summarized in a review truly reflect what can be expected in routine care (Glasziou et al. 1998).

Bringing review findings into clinical practice usually involves a range of techniques to promote, implement, and then maintain change. There are a number of ways to disseminate research findings to investigators and practitioners (Wilson et al. 2001) and guidelines for doing so (NHS Centre for Reviews and Dissemination 1999). According to the Cochrane Collaboration (2007) and Wilson et al. (2001):

- Most interventions are effective under some circumstances, but none is effective under all circumstances;
- Interventions that take potential barriers into account are more likely to be effective;
- Multifaceted interventions that target multiple barriers to change are more likely to be effective than those that target single barriers;
- Reminder systems, such as those for fostering adherence to clinical guidelines, are generally effective for a range of clinician behaviors;
- Audits, feedback from leaders or other authorities, and other techniques have mixed effects and should be used selectively; and
- Educational outreach is generally effective in changing prescribing behavior.

Often, it is not clear why some dissemination techniques work in one setting but not others. Success is more likely when the needs and perceptions of the target group – for example, nurses or physicians – are assessed and satisfied (Wilson et al. 2001). Other factors that warrant consideration before a change in clinical practice takes place include:

- Whether there are sufficient resources, such as time and money for staff training;
- Whether the problem can be solved;

- Whether the professionals who must change the way they practice perceive the problem as significant;
- Whether key stakeholders and personnel are supportive; and
- The extent to which the change is consistent with the organization's policy (NHS Centre for Reviews and Dissemination 1999; Wilson et al. 2001).

Before a change occurs, it is important to gauge the willingness to change, the factors that may influence adoption of the new practice, the preparedness of the targeted professionals to change, potential barriers, and the factors that will enable change, including resources and skills (NHS Centre for Reviews and Dissemination 1999; Wilson et al. 2001).

Practice-based evidence

The EBP model has been criticized for failing to improve clinical practice. One reason it has not achieved this aim is that researchers and practitioners often live in two different worlds. Researchers generate and test ideas, often under controlled conditions, without any connection to the routines of daily care (McDonald & Viehbeck 2007). Results, which usually are presented at academic meetings and in peer-reviewed journals, do not necessarily reach the practitioners who are expected to use them (McDonald & Viehbeck 2007).

Practitioners, meanwhile, are not involved in the research process, may not understand it well, or may lack confidence in the relevance of research to their own practice (Evans et al. 2003). They need relevant information they can easily comprehend and readily apply to their particular setting and patients. They also need techniques for implementing interventions in light of contextual details and practical considerations. Bringing research findings into practice requires attention to basic operational questions; merely creating and disseminating data are not sufficient (McDonald & Viehbeck 2007).

The strong reliance of the EBP paradigm on randomized controlled trials and systematic literature reviews limits the extent to which research findings can be generalized. Such trials often have strict inclusion and exclusion criteria and they either ignore or try to control for variations in clinical practice (Hoagwood et al. 2001; Roy-Byrne et al. 2003; Weisz & Kazdin 2003; Walker & Bruns 2006). While well-controlled efficacy studies are important in determining causation, there has been little attempt to examine interventions under typical and varying, rather than optimal, conditions (Glasgow et al. 2003; Green & Glasgow 2006). This limits studies' relevance to many practice situations and the conclusions that can be drawn from them.

To overcome these barriers, practice-based evidence (PBE) has emerged as an approach that complements EBP. It generates evidence derived from and applicable to routine practice. There are many untapped research problems in clinical practice that need scientifically sound and applicable solutions. Another promising PBE route is research on the effectiveness of interventions in clinical use that have not been rigorously studied.

PBE brings together the best of the researcher and clinician worlds: the expertise of researchers to translate clinical problems into meaningful questions for rigorous investigation, and clinical experts' in-depth knowledge about their practice setting and patients, the interventions they use and why, and what constitutes a meaningful and clinically relevant research problem.

PBE seeks to enhance external validity, or the extent to which findings can be generalized to the larger population, while speeding up the development of valid and effective interventions in an orderly fashion, moving from intervention design to studies of efficacy and effectiveness (Walker & Bruns 2006). Studies derived from clinical practice have high external validity because the interventions they examine are used routinely. However, potentially confounding factors related to large variations in practices and patients may dilute observed effects or make it difficult to explain why a particular result occurs. This drastically reduces a study's internal validity (Audin et al. 2001).

Therefore, two key components of PBE are effectiveness and practice (National Advisory Mental Health Council 1999). Effectiveness refers to the generalizability of results *across* particular services and settings; it addresses external validity. Practice refers to the ability to ascertain results *within* a particular service or setting, taking into account individual differences and variations of patient subgroups; it addresses internal validity. Achieving both external and internal validity is challenging because it requires much larger sample sizes than those usually necessary to establish only effectiveness (Barkham et al. 2001).

Among the models that have emerged to facilitate PBE are practice research networks (Audin et al. 2001; Barkham & Mellor-Clark 2003), also known as communities of practice (McDonald & Viehbeck 2007). They encompass researchers and practitioners who, sharing a common interest in a particular issue or problem, collaborate on investigating it. Unlike formal research, in which data are collected from clinical trials, practice research networks gather real-world data. Practitioners collect and are part owners of the data. The researchers develop large, clinically representative data sets that enable them to maintain both external and internal validity. A network is typically linked to one or more academic centers that can help keep the group up-to-date on recent scientific developments and assist with research methods and analysis. Such an infrastructure links scientific inquiry with practice to deliver clinically rigorous effectiveness research that generates practical applications (Audin et al. 2001).

Evidence-based, shared decision-making between caregivers and patients

A significant amount of evidence suggests that the main causes of clinical errors resulting from sub-optimal practice are lack of adequate information, such as relevant data or misinterpretation of data, and ineffective communication (Gustafson et al. 1999). Patients are the major source of information for appropriate clinical decision-making, and diagnoses often are based on their self-reports. Failure to obtain adequate information from patients about their illness experiences is a primary cause of incorrect or delayed diagnoses, unidentified symptoms and problems, and, consequently, inadequate care (Hayward et al. 2005).

In evidence-based patient care, not including patients' perspectives on their health problems and not including their treatment and care preferences means important evidence is missing. EBP information alone, which is primarily about whether or not interventions are generally effective, often is insufficient to inform optimal care for individual patients. Clinicians and patients frequently must make difficult decisions in cases where outcomes are uncertain and there are several treatment options. However, clinical evidence regarding the effectiveness of one treatment versus another often does not point to the best option, the stakes may be high, or the treatment decision is associated with a range of strong personal values (O'Connor et al. 1998a, 1998b). For example, patients may have to decide whether they should undergo genetic testing for breast cancer, have a mastectomy or lumpectomy, or undergo prenatal testing. The outcomes of such decisions can have important personal consequences. Clinical decisions also may involve trade-offs, such as quality of life versus length of life, or accepting short-term risks to achieve long-term benefits. Surgery for coronary artery disease, for example, can increase long-term survival at the risk of short-term surgical complications or even death.

Clinical decisions in these situations need to be informed not only by the best available evidence about the effectiveness of interventions, but also by benefits and risks, and treatment alternatives. Because benefits, risks, and aspects of health have different value and meaning to different patients, no single choice is universally correct. In each situation, the pros and cons must be weighed in light of the patient's values, patient preferences must be considered, and implementing the decision must be possible (Hope 2000). Safe clinical decisions in cases of uncertain or value-sensitive outcomes require shared decision-making by caregivers and patients.

Biomedical ethics has long recognized the right of individuals to make decisions about risks to their own life or well-being (Beauchamp & Childress 1983). The concept of shared decision-making capitalizes on the need to modify treatment and care so they meet the patient's values and experiences. Patients help make treatment or screening decisions that are informed by the best available evidence about options and potential benefits and harms, and that consider patient preferences (O'Connor et al. 1999a, 1999b; Molenaar et al. 2000; Holmes-Rovner et al. 2001). Clinicians who fail to obtain patients' perspective can jeopardize achievement of desired outcomes and patient safety.

In recent years, there has been rapid development of decision aids to support shared decision-making – tools, models, methods, and evaluation strategies for eliciting patient preferences. The primary purpose of these aids is to help people make specific and deliberate choices among options by providing, at a minimum, evidence-based information about the options and outcomes relevant to their health status (O'Connor et al. 1999a). In addition, decision aids often help patients personalize this information, understand the inherent uncertainties associated with the choice they make, assist them in clarifying and communicating their values or desires regarding potential benefits relative to potential harms, and prepare them for collaborative decision-making (Elwyn et al. 2006). Among the various decision aid formats are audio-guided workbooks (O'Connor et al. 1999c) and computerized tools such as interactive videodiscs (Barry et al. 1995; Lenert & Soetikno 1997), palm-top applications (Ruland 1999; Ruland et al. 2003), and web-based applications (Lenert 2000; Gustafson et al. 2001, 2002; Lenert & Sturley 2002).[7]

Decision aids are adjuncts to clinical counseling. Patients can use them to prepare for a discussion with their clinician, or clinicians may offer them during a visit to facilitate shared decision-making. There is compelling evidence that decision aids are superior to standard counseling. According to a Cochrane Collaboration review regarding their effectiveness and feasibility, the aids improve patient knowledge, realistic expectations, participation in decision-making, and agreement between patients' values and treatment choice, and they reduce decisional conflict (O'Connor et al. 2001, 2003). Decision aids can also improve treatment uptake and in some cases reduce the use of medical procedures (Elwyn et al. 2006).

More than 500 decision aids produced by non-profit or commercial organizations are now available, many on the Internet. To ensure that the aids are evidence-based and founded on reliable information, the International Patient Decision Aids Standards Collaboration, a group of worldwide researchers, practitioners, and stakeholders, has developed internationally approved quality criteria[8] (Elwyn et al. 2006).

Evidence-based symptom management

Decision aids have been primarily targeted to the relatively narrow segment of decisions about single episodes of screening or treatment choices. Much less work has been carried out on helping clinicians elicit evidence about patients' illness experiences and preferences, and integrating the evidence into management of chronic illness.

Patients with chronic conditions often experience wide-ranging physical, functional, and psychosocial symptoms and problems that clinicians must attend to simultaneously. For example, a patient with congestive obstructive pulmonary disorder may have dyspnea, fatigue, reduced activity, mucus, infections, stress, depression, anxiety, nutritional problems, and other debilitating conditions. In managing chronic illness, a major task is identifying and addressing multiple problems in a manner that gives priority to those that are the most distressing for, and of most concern to, the patient. Because of large individual variations in symptom characteristics (Reilly et al. 1997; Miaskowski 2006), clinicians cannot automatically anticipate what symptoms and problems patients are experiencing or what type of care is in their best interest. Therefore, clinicians could benefit from systems for use at the point of care that help them quickly identify symptoms, problems, and concerns from the patient's perspective, that support effective patient–provider communication, and that help clinicians select appropriate evidence-based interventions tailored to each patient's needs.

CHOICE, an acronym for Creating better Health Outcomes by Improving Communication about patients' Experiences, is an interactive computer application designed for this purpose. It guides patients through a systematic self-assessment of symptoms, problems, and concerns, including symptom distress and patients' priorities for care. After the assessment, CHOICE creates a summary that ranks symptoms according to those priorities. Together, clinicians and patients can use the summary to develop a care plan immediately.

Ruland et al. (2006) found that CHOICE elicited significantly more symptoms and that there was significantly greater congruence between patients' reported symptoms and those their clinician addressed. Using CHOICE also resulted in better achievement of patient-preferred outcomes, better functional status, and higher patient satisfaction (Ruland 1999, 2002).

A university hospital in Norway has successfully integrated the CHOICE application into standard care on several cancer units. This has generated a number of exciting new research opportunities and illustrates how evidence-based practice can move to the next step: practice-based evidence. Using CHOICE to obtain clinical data from all patients in these units generates large data sets that satisfy the need for internal and external validity, the key components of PBE. In addition, these data sets enable researchers to study the effects of CHOICE under different practice conditions and in subgroups of patients with various cancer diagnoses, stages of disease, or demographic characteristics. A practice research network comprising clinical practice nurses and investigators will determine how to successfully integrate the application into routine health care practice.

Evidence-based self-management of illness

While the EBP literature focuses primarily on supporting clinicians at the point of care, patients – particularly those with chronic illnesses – mostly manage their illness alone at home, unsupervised by health care professionals. Additionally, the side effects of treatment often are the most severe after discharge from the hospital; many patients experience considerable symptom distress without much assistance. A major barrier to safe patient care and effective symptom management is the limited availability of evidence-based, self-management support for patients.

Widespread use of the Internet offers unique opportunities to support patients with evidence-based information specific to their needs. In many countries, empowering patients to have a more active role in their health and giving them access to reliable information are high-priority health policy goals. A patient who thoroughly understands his or her diagnosis, treatment, and recovery, and who has support from others, is much better equipped to manage illness, to change health-related behaviors, and to use the health care system more effectively (Gallienne et al. 1993; Brennan 1997; Gustafson et al. 1999; Moore et al. 2001; Fleisher et al. 2002). Brennan et al. (2001) demonstrated that people of all ages, even if they are computer novices, use web-based technology to obtain health information, peer support, and professional assistance. However, the overwhelming volume of health-related information online and its often questionable quality mean patients need help finding information that is specific, reliable, and useful.

Internet applications enable information to be tailored to the needs of individual patients. Tailored messages are more effective than the 'one size fits all' approach of many educational or information sources because they are more personally relevant. Furthermore, people can better understand and remember such messages and thus are more likely to change their behavior (Kreuter et al. 1999). Tailoring is particularly important for chronically ill patients, as symptom distress varies widely among patients and can change during different illness stages or even from day to day.

Conclusions

Although bringing evidence into practice remains a challenge, there are feasible ways to accomplish this important task. Among them are including patients as an additional source of evidence to improve clinical decision-making, generating evidence from practice, and, via information technology, supporting symptom self-management with evidence where and when patients need it.

Developing such technology is complex. It requires a synthesis of knowledge from numerous domains, including clinical research, behavioral change, and medical informatics, which provides the tools and algorithms to collect, process, structure, present, and integrate evidence into patient care. It also requires organizational knowledge. Organizations must be able to adapt evidence to clinical practice and workflow, and to their unique professional context.

Notes

1 www.cochranelibrary.com
2 www.tripdatabase.com
3 sumsearch.uthscsa.edu
4 www.crd.york.ac.uk/crdweb
5 clinicalevidence.bmj.com/ceweb/index.jsp
6 www.nice.org.uk
7 An excellent source for decision aids is the Ottawa Decision Support Framework (decisionaid.ohri.ca/methods.html). These aids integrate concepts and theories related to general and social psychology, decision analysis, decisional conflict, social support, and self-efficacy (Ottawa Health Research Institute 2007).
8 Available at decisionaid.ohri.ca/methods.html#checklist.

References

Audin, K., Mellor-Clark, J., Barkham, M., Margison, F., McGrath, G., Lewis, S., et al. (2001) Practice research networks for effective psychological therapies. *Journal of Mental Health* **10**(3), 241–251.

Barkham, M., Margison, F., Leach, C., Lucock, M., Mellor-Clark, J., Evans, C., et al. (2001) Service profiling and outcomes benchmarking using the CORE-OM: Toward practice-based evidence in the psychological therapies. *Journal of Consulting and Clinical Psychology* **69**(2), 184–196.

Barkham, M. & Mellor-Clark, J. (2003) Bridging evidence-based practice and practice-based evidence: Developing a rigorous and relevant knowledge for the psychological therapies. *Clinical Psychology & Psychotherapy* **10**(6), 319–327.

Barry, M.J., Fowler, F.J. Jr., Mulley, A.G. Jr., Henderson, J.V. Jr. & Wennberg, J.E. (1995) Patient reactions to a program designed to facilitate patient participation in treatment decisions for benign prostatic hyperplasia. *Medical Care* **33**(8), 771–782.

Beauchamp, T.L. & Childress, J.F. (1983) *Principles of biomedical ethics*, 2nd Edn. New York: Oxford University Press.

Brennan, P.F. (1997) The ComputerLink projects: A decade of experience. *Studies in Health Technology and Informatics* **46**, 521–526.

Brennan, P.F., Moore, S.M., Bjornsdottir, G., Jones, J., Visovsky, C. & Rogers, M. (2001) HeartCare: An Internet-based information and support system for patient home recovery after coronary artery bypass graft (CABG) surgery. *Journal of Advanced Nursing* **35**(5), 699–708.

Chalmers, I. & Altmann, D. (1995) *Systematic reviews*. London: BMJ Publishing Group.

Cochrane Collaboration (2007) Cochrane Effective Practice and Organisation of Care Group. Ottawa: Cochrane Collaboration. Available at www.epoc.cochrane.org/en/index.html.

Degner, L.F. & Sloan, J.A. (1992) Decision making during serious illness: What role do patients really want to play? *Journal of Clinical Epidemiology* **45**(9), 941–950.

Elwyn, G., O'Connor, A., Stacey, D., Volk, R., Edwards, A., Coulter, A., et al., International Patient Decision Aids Standards Collaboration (2006) Developing a quality criteria framework for patient decision aids: Online international Delphi consensus process. *British Medical Journal* **333**(7565), 417.

Evans, C., Connell, J., Barkham, M., Marshall, C. & Mellor-Clark, J. (2003) Practice-based evidence: Benchmarking NHS primary care counselling services at national and local levels. *Clinical Psychology & Psychotherapy* **10**(6), 374–388.

Fleisher, L., Bass, S., Ruzek, S.B. & McKeown-Conn, N. (2002) Relationships among Internet health information use, patient behavior and self efficacy in newly diagnosed cancer patients who contact the National Cancer Institute's NCI Atlantic Region Cancer Information Service (CIS). *AMIA Annual Symposium Proceedings* (pp. 260–264).

Gallienne, R.L., Moore, S.M. & Brennan, P.F. (1993) Alzheimer's caregivers: Psychosocial support via computer networks. *Journal of Gerontology Nursing* **19**(12), 15–22.

Glasgow, R.E., Lichtenstein, E. & Marcus, A.C. (2003) Why don't we see more translation of health promotion research to practice? Rethinking the efficacy-to-effectiveness transition. *American Journal of Public Health* **93**(8), 1261–1267.

Glasziou, P., Guyatt, G., Dans, A., Dans, L., Straus, S. & Sackett, D. (1998) Applying the results of trials and systematic reviews to individual patients. *Evidence Based Medicine* **3**, 165–166.

Green, L.W. & Glasgow, R.E. (2006) Evaluating the relevance, generalization, and applicability of research: Issues in external validation and translation methodology. *Evaluation & the Health Professions* **29**(1), 126–153.

Gustafson, D., Hawkins, R., Boberg, E., McTavish, F., Owens, B., Wise, M., et al. (2002) CHESS: 10 years of research and development in consumer health informatics for broad populations, including the underserved. *International Journal of Medical Informatics* **65**(3), 169–177.

Gustafson, D.H., Hawkins, R., Boberg, E., Pingree, S., Serlin, R.E., Graziano, F., et al. (1999) Impact of a patient-centered, computer-based health information/support system. *American Journal of Preventive Medicine* **16**(1), 1–9.

Gustafson, D., Hawkins, R., Pingree, S., McTavish, F., Arora, N., Mendenhall, J., et al. (2001) Effect of computer support on younger women with breast cancer. *Journal of Internal Medicine* **16**(7), 435–445.

Haines, A. & Donald, A. (2002) Introduction. In A. Haines, A. Donald (Eds) *Getting research findings into practice*, 2nd Edn (pp. 1–10). London: BMJ Publishing Group.

Hayward, R.A., Asch, S.M., Hogan, M.M., Hofer, T.P. & Kerr, E.A. (2005) Sins of omission: Getting too little medical care may be the greatest threat to patient safety. *Journal of General Internal Medicine* **20**(8), 686–691.

Hoagwood, K., Burns, B.J., Kiser, L., Ringeisen, H. & Schoenwald, S.K. (2001) Evidence-based practice in child and adolescent mental health services. *Psychiatric Services* **52**(9), 1179–1189.

Holmes-Rovner, M., Llewellyn-Thomas, H., Entwistle, V., Coulter, A., O'Connor, A. & Rovner, D.R. (2001) Patient choice modules for summaries of clinical effectiveness: A proposal. *British Medical Journal* **322**(7287), 664–667.

Holmes-Rovner, M., Valade, D., Orlowski, C., Draus, C., Nabozny-Valerio, B. & Keiser, S. (2000) Implementing shared decision-making in routine practice: Barriers and opportunities. *Health Expectations* **3**(3), 182–191.

Hope, T. (2000) *Evidence-based patient choice*. London: Kings Fund Publishing.

Kreuter, M.W., Bull, F.C., Clark, E.M. & Oswald, D.L. (1999) Understanding how people process health information: A comparison of tailored and nontailored weight-loss materials. *Health Psychology* **18**(5), 487–494.

Lenert, L.A. (2000) iMPACT3: Online tools for development of Web sites for the study of patients' preferences and utilities. *AMIA Annual Symposium Proceedings* 1172.

Lenert, L.A. & Soetikno, R.M. (1997) Automated computer interviews to elicit utilities: Potential applications in the treatment of deep venous thrombosis. *Journal of the American Medical Informatics Association* **4**(1), 49–56.

Lenert, L.A. & Sturley, A.E. (2002) Use of the Internet to study the utility values of the public. *AMIA Annual Symposium Proceedings* 440–444.

McDonald, P.W. & Viehbeck, S. (2007) From evidence-based practice making to practice-based evidence making: Creating communities of (research) and practice. *Health Promotion Practice* **8**(2), 140–144.

Miaskowski, C. (2006) Symptom clusters: Establishing the link between clinical practice and symptom management research. *Supportive Care in Cancer* **14**(8), 792–794.

Molenaar, S., Sprangers, M.A., Postma-Schuit, F.C., Rutgers, E.J., Noorlander, J., Hendriks, J., et al. (2000) Feasibility and effects of decision aids. *Medical Decision Making* **20**(1), 112–127.

Moore, S.M., Brennan, P.F., O'Brien, R., Visovsky, C. & Bjornsdottir, G. (2001) Customized computer home support improves recovery of CABG patients. *Circulation* **104**(2 Suppl), II533.

National Advisory Mental Health Council (1999) *Bridging science and service: A report by the National Advisory Mental Health Council's Clinical Treatment and Services Research Workshop*, Report No. 99-4353. Washington, D.C: National Institute of Mental Health.

NHS Centre for Reviews and Dissemination (1999) Getting evidence into practice. *Effective Health Care* **5**(1), 1–16.

O'Connor, A.M., Drake, E.R., Fiset, V., Graham, I.D., Laupacis, A. & Tugwell, P. (1999c) The Ottawa patient decision aids. *Effective Clinical Practice* **2**(4), 163–170.

O'Connor, A.M., Fiset, V., DeGrasse, C., Graham, I.D., Evans, W., Stacey, D., et al. (1999b) Decision aids for patients considering options affecting cancer outcomes: Evidence of efficacy and policy implications. *Journal of the National Cancer Institute Monographs* **25**, 67–80.

O'Connor, A.M., Rostom, A., Fiset, V., Tetroe, J., Entwistle, V., Llewellyn-Thomas, H., et al. (1999a) Decision aids for patients facing health treatment or screening decisions: Systematic review. *British Medical Journal* **319**(7212), 731–734.

O'Connor, A.M., Stacey, D., Entwistle, V., Llewellyn-Thomas, H., Rovner, D., Holmes-Rovner, M., et al. (2003) Decision aids for people facing health treatment or screening decisions. *Cochrane Database of Systematic Reviews* CD001431.

O'Connor, A.M., Stacey, D., Rovner, D., Holmes-Rovner, M., Tetroe, J., Llewellyn-Thomas, H., et al. (2001) Decision aids for people facing health treatment or screening decisions. *Cochrane Database of Systematic Reviews* CD001431.

O'Connor, A.M., Tugwell, P., Wells, G.A., Elmslie, T., Jolly, E., Hollingworth, G., et al. (1998a) A decision aid for women considering hormone therapy after menopause: Decision support framework and evaluation. *Patient Education and Counseling* **33**(3), 267–279.

O'Connor, A.M., Tugwell, P., Wells, G.A., Elmslie, T., Jolly, E., Hollingworth, G., et al. (1998b) Randomized trial of a portable, self-administered decision aid for post-menopausal women considering long-term preventive hormone therapy. *Medical Decision Making* **18**(3), 295–303.

Ottawa Health Research Institute (2006) Ottawa decision support framework to address decisional conflict. Ottawa: Ottawa Health Research Institute. Available at www.decisionaid.ohri.ca/docs/develop/ODSF.pdf.

Reilly, C.A., Holzemer, W.L., Henry, S.B., Slaughter, R.E. & Portillo, C.J. (1997) A comparison of patient and nurse ratings of human immunodeficiency virus-related signs and symptoms. *Nursing Research* **46**(6), 318–323.

Roy-Byrne, P.P., Sherbourne, C.D., Craske, M.G., Stein, M.B., Katon, W., Sullivan, G., et al. (2003) Moving treatment research from clinical trials to the real world. *Psychiatric Services* **54**(3), 327–332.

Ruland, C., Røislien, J., Bakken, S. & Kristiansen, J. (2006) Comparing tailored computerized symptom assessments to interviews and questionnaires. Annual Symposium of the American Medical Informatics Association. Washington, D.C.: November 11–15.

Ruland, C.M. (1999) Decision support for patient preference-based care planning: Effects on nursing care and patient outcomes. *Journal of the American Medical Informatics Association* **6**(4), 304–312.

Ruland, C.M. (2002) Handheld technology to improve patient care: Evaluating a support system for preference-based care planning at the bedside. *Journal of the American Medical Informatics Association* **9**(2), 192–201.

Ruland, C.M. (2005) CHOICEs: Patients as participants in shared care planning at the point of care. In D. Lewis, G. Eysenbach, R. Kukafka, P.Z. Stavri & H.B. Jimison (Eds) *Consumer health informatics: informing consumers and improving health care* (pp. 208–216). New York: Springer.

Ruland, C.M., White, T., Stevens, M., Fanciullo, G. & Khilani, S.M. (2003) Effects of a computerized system to support shared decision making in symptom management of cancer patients: Preliminary results. *Journal of the American Medical Informatics Association* **10**(6), 573–579.

Walker, J.S. & Bruns, E.J. (2006) Building on practice-based evidence: Using expert perspectives to define the wraparound process. *Psychiatric Services* **57**(11), 1579–1585.

Weisz, J.R. & Kazdin, A.E. (2003) Concluding thoughts: Present and future of evidence-based psychotherapies for children and adolescents. In A.E. Kazdin & J.R. Weisz (Eds) *Evidence-based psychotherapies for children and adolescents* (pp. 439–451). New York: Guilford Press.

Wilson, P., Richardson, R., Sowden, A.J. & Evans, D. (2001) *Stage III. Reporting and dissemination. Phase 9. Getting evidence into practice.* York, UK: NHS Centre for Reviews and Dissemination.

Index